BEYOND THE BOX: B.F. SKINNER'S TECHNOLOGY OF BEHAVIOR FROM LABORATORY TO LIFE, 1950s–1970s

B.F. Skinner (1904–1990) is one of the most famous and influential figures in twentieth-century psychology. A best-selling author, inventor, and social commentator, Skinner was both a renowned scientist and a public intellectual known for his controversial theories of human behavior. *Beyond the Box* is the first full-length study of the ways in which Skinner's ideas left the laboratory to become part of the post-war public's everyday lives, and chronicles both the enthusiasm and caution with which this process was received.

Using selected case studies, Alexandra Rutherford provides a fascinating account of Skinner and his acolytes' attempts to weave their technology of human behavior into the politically turbulent fabric of 1950s to 1970s American life. To detail their innovative methods, Rutherford uses extensive archival materials and interviews to study the Skinnerians' creation of human behavior laboratories, management programs for juvenile delinquents, psychiatric wards, and prisons, as well as their influence on the self-help industry with popular books on how to quit smoking, lose weight, and be more assertive.

A remarkable look at a post-war scientific and technological revolution, *Beyond the Box* is a rewarding study of how behavioral theories met real-life problems, and the ways in which Skinner and his followers continue to influence the present.

ALEXANDRA RUTHERFORD is an associate professor in the Department of Psychology at York University.

Beyond the Box

B.F. Skinner's Technology of Behavior from Laboratory to Life, 1950s–1970s

Alexandra Rutherford

UNIVERSITY OF TORONTO PRESS
Toronto Buffalo London

© University of Toronto Press Incorporated 2009
Toronto Buffalo London
www.utppublishing.com
Printed in Canada

ISBN 978-0-8020-9774-3 (cloth)
ISBN 978-0-8020-9618-0 (paper)

Printed on acid-free paper

Library and Archives Canada Cataloguing in Publication

Rutherford, Alexandra, 1971–
    Beyond the box: B. F. Skinnner's technology of behavior
from laboratory to life, 1950s–1970s / Alexandra Rutherford.

    Includes index.
    ISBN 978-0-8020-9774-3 (bound)   ISBN 978-0-8020-9618-0 (pbk.)

    1. Skinner, B. F. (Burrhus Frederic), 1904–1990.   2. Behaviorism
(Psychology).   I. Title.

    BF199.R88 2009   150.19'434092   C2008-907708-3

University of Toronto Press acknowledges the financial assistance to its publishing program of the Canada Council for the Arts and the Ontario Arts Council.

University of Toronto Press acknowledges the financial support for its publishing activities of the Government of Canada through the Book Publishing Industry Development Program (BPIDP).

This book has been published with the help of a grant from the Canadian Federation for the Humanities and Social Sciences, through the Aid to Scholarly Publications Program, using funds provided by the Social Sciences and Humanities Research Council of Canada.

Contents

Acknowledgments

I began my acquaintance with B.F. Skinner and the technology of behavior during my doctoral studies in the History and Theory of Psychology graduate program at York University in Toronto. I am now privileged to be a tenured faculty member in that program. Skinner played no small part in helping bring that about. So first, my thanks go to B.F. Skinner for providing me with a rich subject of scholarship and research, and to his followers for accepting me into their ranks so hospitably over the past several years. In the course of researching this book, I have attended and participated in behavior analytic conferences both large and intimate, cultivated relationships with behavior analysts throughout the United States, Canada, Central America, and Europe, made a short visit to Twin Oaks in beautiful Louisa, Virginia, and have of course spent extended periods of time in the B.F. Skinner Papers at the Harvard University Archives in Cambridge, Massachusetts.

Cambridge was Skinner's stomping ground both as a graduate student and, after brief stints in Minnesota and Indiana, again as a Harvard faculty member for most of his career. Although the Harvard Pigeon Lab is now a fading memory in the minds of those who inhabited the basement warren of Memorial Hall, and Skinner himself has not graced the corridors of William James Hall for almost two decades, I could not resist trying to evoke the feeling of that pioneering time in my frequent visits to Cambridge over the past several years.

During my idle moments between interviews and archives grubbing, I popped into the Sheraton Commander and imagined Fred Skinner and Fred Keller meeting up for a vodka and tonic at the end of the day, sharing news and gossip, or planning their next experiments. I had the opportunity to visit Skinner's house on Old Dee Road during a reception hosted by his daughter Dr Julie Vargas and her husband, Ernest. Although the pool was covered over for the winter (or had perhaps been filled in, I cannot quite recall), one could almost imagine Skinner and his two young daughters splashing merrily in the water on a hot mid-summer afternoon. I attended a concert at Sanders Theater in Memorial Hall, mostly, I'll admit, to wander through the basement during intermission, hoping to find some vestige of the once-vaunted Pigeon Lab – a feather, perhaps, or a pellet – but discovered instead a gorgeously renovated Student Commons, not a feather to be found.

However, Skinner – as I point out at the beginning of this account – is not the main subject of this work. I could instead have attempted to find the vestiges of Harold Cohen's CASE project at the National Training School for Boys in Washington, DC, a city which was home to me for a substantial period of time while working on this book. I was unsuccessful, however, in locating either Harold Cohen's current whereabouts, or the site of the former National Training School, which I assume has long since been redeveloped. Neither could I visit the abandoned hydrotherapy unit in the basement of Metropolitan State Hospital in Waltham, Massachusetts, where Ogden Lindsley constructed his Skinner-box rooms for the Behavior Research Laboratory. The hospital was closed in 1991 and the site slated for demolition and redevelopment.

But as I have argued throughout this account, Skinner's technology of behavior, as rooted as it was in work that took place in particular places and precise physical spaces, has managed to transcend its places of provenance. Witness the extremely well attended annual meetings of the Association for Behavior Analysis International. In the meeting spaces, banquet halls, and ballrooms of the large hotels where the convention meets, you will find Skinner's spirit embodied in the thousands of Skinnerian psychologists and practitioners using his principles throughout the country and around the world. It was at these conferences that I met many of the people who have contributed to this book, either by imparting their knowledge and perspectives, introducing me to important contacts, including me in conference programs, inviting me to give talks, lending or giving me materials, or simply allowing me to bend their ears with questions about behavior analysis. Several of these people agreed to sit for recorded interviews, providing me with material that was directly used in the manuscript or indirectly informed my understanding of behavior analysis. For their generosity of time, I am extremely grateful. They are: Julie Skinner Vargas, Jack Michael, Teodoro Ayllon, the late Ogden Lindsley, Scott Geller, Jackson Marr, Edward Morris,

Joseph Pear, Joseph Morrow, and James Holland. I would like to single out Jack Michael and Scott Geller for special thanks. They were both an ongoing help throughout this project, and were most generous in sharing their memories and materials, including photos.

I am also indebted to the late Beatrice Barrett, who spoke with me at length by phone about her work at the Fernald State School and directed me to several important resources for understanding the role of measurement in applied behavior analysis. The late W. Scott Wood was another source of constant support, encouragement, and enthusiasm for preserving the history of behavior analysis, and gave me his copy of the Drake Conference proceedings, which helped immeasurably with chapter 4. Peter Nathan, who did a postdoctoral fellowship at Ogden Lindsley's Behavior Research Laboratory from 1962 to 1964, shared information about his time at the laboratory and directed me to further publications. Nancy Hughes Lindsley was extremely generous in locating, scanning, and sharing photos from the Ogden Lindsley Archive.

Stephanie Tomiyasu (formerly Stolz) was invaluable in pointing me towards her materials at the Archives of the History of American Psychology and answering my questions about her time on the APA Commission on Behavior Modification. Victor Laties gave me material from his personal collection and educated me about behavioral pharmacology. John Mabry likewise shared personal materials and remembrances from the very early days of applied behavior analysis. Carol Pilgrim shared information about the experimental analysis of human behavior, and Gerald Shook provided me with materials and information about certification for behavior analysts.

Among my non-behavior analytic informers was Barbara Mishkin, one of the staff members of the National Commission for the Protection of Human Subjects of Biomedical and Behavioral Research, who allowed me to come to her law office and photocopy her personal materials and documents from the Commission. Many thanks to her and her insights about this important work. David Clark shared his personal correspondence with Eileen Allen, which helped flesh out my understanding of Bijou's work and influence at the University of Washington. The late Kat Kinkade responded patiently to my e-mail requests for information on what must have seemed to her like well-traversed terrain. And just to show that Skinner is indeed everywhere, thanks to Marguerite Bouvard, who during my stay at the Brandeis Women's Studies Research Center to do research for another, unrelated project, shared with me her experience at Twin Oaks and gave me a copy of her book on intentional communities, which I cite in chapter 6.

I also benefitted enormously from my association with the International Society for Behaviorology, where conversations with David Palmer, Phil Hineline, Robert Allan, Julie and Ernest Vargas, Joseph Morrow, and Jerome Ulman were particularly stimulating. Special thanks go to Joseph Morrow and Jerome Ulman for sharing their experiences with and materials about Behaviorists for Social Action, which will be another chapter in another book!

Of special note for helping me keep Skinner and behaviorism in perspective, and for his enthusiastic proofreading of the manuscript, is Clive Wynne. His excitement about the project has also helped me see it through to its conclusion. My colleague Andrew Winston, a fine historian of psychology, has also contributed to my understanding of radical behaviorism and its history and context. Of extra-special note is Edward Morris, who has been enormously helpful and supportive over many years, generously sharing his knowledge, expertise, and resources on all things behavior-analytic. Ed has put in countless hours of reviewing on my behalf when an expert on the history of behavior analysis was needed to evaluate my work, and carefully proofread this manuscript despite his own massively busy schedule. His scholarly contributions and collegiality have helped me understand behavior analysis and history in myriad ways. He has also facilitated important contacts and been my guide in navigating the scientific and professional world of behavior analysis. Without his help, this book could not have been written. Any infelicities or inaccuracies that remain in this manuscript are, however, mine and mine alone.

Although we have had fewer informal conversations, Laurence Smith's published work on Skinner and the technological imperative has been an invaluable resource to me for its richness of analysis and depth of understanding. Finally, I also extend my appreciation to Raymond Fancher, who has always been a staunch supporter of me and my scholarship, and is a model writer and historian of psychology. It is a privilege to have him as my mentor, and I look forward to working with him for many years to come.

Portions of this work have been published and presented in numerous venues over the past several years, including the Society for the History of Psychology meetings at the American Psychological Association annual conventions, the meetings of Cheiron, the International Society for the History of the Behavioral and Social Sciences, and the History of Science Society convention. Portions of chapters 1 and 4 have been previously published in the *Journal of the History of the Behavioral Sciences* (see Rutherford, 2003, 2006), copyright © Wiley Periodicals, Inc. Numerous archivists have been extremely helpful over the course of many visits, especially the staff at the Harvard University Archives and the Archives of the History of American Psychology (AHAP). AHAP's Lizette Royer, Reference Archivist, Dorothy Gruich, Senior Archivist, and David Baker, Director of Archives, have all been infinitely helpful and amazingly hospitable.

The writing of this book would not have been possible without the support of a Faculty of Arts Research Fellowship from York University, which granted me the time for travel and research without the constraints of teaching and administration. A Social Sciences and Humanities Research Council of Canada Standard Research Grant provided much-needed financial support for travel, archival work, and research assistance during four years of the book's incubation and development. I thank my editor at University of Toronto Press, Lennart Husband, for being willing to take a chance on an unknown author with an interesting topic. I would also like to thank Tera Beaulieu for her absolutely expert assistance in formatting and proofreading the manuscript.

My biggest thanks and most ardent appreciation, however, go to my partner in love and work, Wade Edward Pickren. As an accomplished historian of psychology, his advice, perspective, and support have been expert, well informed, and gratifying. Having his wealth of knowledge about the history of American psychology consistently at my disposal has been an absolutely wondrous gift. As my partner in life, his unwavering faith in my ability, his gracious willingness to alter his career path to accommodate mine, and his incredible generosity of spirit buoy and amaze me at all times. His ability to make me laugh, and all the laughs we have shared, make our life together a constant source of pleasure and release. It is to Wade that I lovingly dedicate this book.

BEYOND THE BOX: B.F. SKINNER'S TECHNOLOGY
OF BEHAVIOR FROM LABORATORY TO LIFE, 1950s–1970s

Introduction: Beyond the Box

He's a legend in his time. He's a loaded subject. His ideas about control and manipulation have been called evil. He has been accused of setting back the study of psychology rather than advancing it. He has also been called one of the most incisive thinkers of modern times.

Sanford, 1977, p. 21

One of the conspicuous features of B.F. Skinner's life and work is the contrast between the cautious experimental research that brought him recognition as a laboratory scientist and the expansive social philosophy that later brought him wider renown. Indeed, Skinner's call for the redesign of culture on the basis of experiments with lower organisms in contrived environments has struck many of his critics as presumptuous or even bizarre.

Smith, 1996a, p. 56

Presumptuous, bizarre – relatively mild epithets in the context of behaviorist B.F. Skinner's controversial career. For the views he expressed in his 1971 *New York Times* best-seller *Beyond Freedom and Dignity*,[1] he was characterized as a 'fatuous opinionated ass,' an 'apologist for totalitarianism,'[2] and 'visibly insane'[3] by incensed readers. So how did the cautious experimentalist, mild-mannered Harvard psychologist, inveterate gadgeteer,[4] lover of Thoreau, and doting father of two come to incite such ire in his audiences? And how can we reconcile the visceral reactions of his critics with those who heralded him as one of the most incisive thinkers of modern times?

For the last several years, I have attempted to answer this question by analyzing B.F. Skinner's transformation from laboratory scientist to public intellectual against the backdrop of mid-twentieth-century American life and the emergence of a psychological society (see Rutherford, 2000, 2003, 2004). I have proposed that popular reactions to Skinner were far more nuanced than typical accounts have suggested, and that these highly varying responses could be understood only with reference to the divergent cultural, historical, and political discourses that informed them. That is, to make sense of the often contradictory portrayals of Skinner in the popular imagination, we needed to understand the popular imagination itself. Further, I have argued that the perceived social and ideological import of his system has been more important for his public image than whether his claims about human behavior were scientifically supported or the applications of his work were verifiably effective. In the realm of public opinion, whether Skinner was 'correct' about human nature – or at least about human *behavior* – was less important than what his system implied for how Americans should view themselves.

As one of America's most famous psychologists, and arguably one of the most prominent scientists of the past century, Skinner played a decisive role in shaping psychological society in the twentieth century. He not only influenced images of psychological science in the popular imagination, he also confronted and attacked many of the highly entrenched views individuals held of themselves and the society in which they lived. His iconoclasm engendered intense popular reaction and earned him a prominent place in popular culture. Skinnerian themes and inventions (if not Skinner himself) turned up in cartoons, science fair projects, Dewar's whiskey ads, and the pages of *Playboy* (see Pearce, 1972; Yafa, 1973). Skinner's legacy continues to influence images of psychology in the popular imagination. Moreover, the cultural, social, and political discourses of mid-twentieth-century American life shaped popular representations of Skinner, and his work, in multiple and complex ways.

To understand Skinner's unique role in the interplay between psychology and its publics, it is important to consider the social and disciplinary contexts in which psychological ideas were both produced and received during the years of his career. Skinner lived and worked in a century marked by an unprecedented awareness of the psychological, an era in which psychology was used as a way to understand and organize personal and interpersonal experience, as well as society. As Roger Smith (1997) has written:

It became possible to refer to the existence of 'psychological society' in the twentieth century ... [T]here is a significant sense in which everyone in the twentieth century learned to be a psychologist; everyone became her or his own psychologist, able and willing to describe life in psychological terms. (R. Smith, pp. 575, 577)

Smith's 'psychological society' refers to a society newly cognizant of the organized discipline of psychology, a discipline claiming expert knowledge of human nature and the specialized techniques with which to measure or modify it. Burnham (1987) has noted that 'for much of the nineteenth century it was not possible to popularize psychology. What psychology there was, was common property among educated people' (p. 85). It was not until the turn of the century that 'specialized, distinctive, scientific psychology came along' (p. 85).

Thus, with the advent of scientific psychology in America in the late 1800s, an area previously unconsolidated and unclaimed by any one professional group – the study of human psychological processes – was taken up by specialists. These specialists claimed that with their new instruments and objective methods, they could shed light on people's thoughts and feelings, reveal new insights into human nature, and lay bare the structure of the soul. Rose (1992) has referred to this as the rise of the 'calculability of the person,' involving the genesis not simply of a new kind of organized knowledge, but of a new rubric of self- and other-construal. Early popularizers of the new psychology made appeals to the public to recognize the scientific, and therefore privileged, status of the new discipline (e.g., Jastrow, 1889; Ruckmich, 1918). In addition, they attempted to persuade the public of the usefulness of their new science by offering prescriptions in almost every area of life, from how to raise well-adjusted children (Watson, 1928) to how to keep mentally fit (Jastrow, 1928).

The assimilation of scientific psychological discourse and its products into the fabric of American society signaled a subtle but noticeable shift in the way the public regarded themselves and their subjective worlds:

The internalization of belief in psychological knowledge ... altered everyone's subjective world and recreated experience and expectations about what it is to be a person. The result was an emphasis on 'the personal' in psychological terms, with ramifications in every aspect of life. (R. Smith, 1997, p. 575)

Newly conscious of 'the personal,' members of this society were eager to hear insights from experts in this new area of professional endeavor, experts whom, they were asked to believe, possessed no less than a 'microscope for the soul' (Hall, 1901, as cited in Burnham, 1987). Although a version of psychology that made no distinction between public and expert had certainly existed before the discipline was formally organized, the 'new psychology' distinguished itself by bringing the naturalism and materialism of the physical sciences to bear on its subject matter. In a sentiment that would later echo loudly in reactions to Skinner's work, some critics of the 'new psychology' claimed that it was 'psychology without a soul.' They argued that the tools of natural science, such as quantification and objective measurement, were hopelessly inappropriate for psychology's subject matter. The public, for their part, were not altogether certain how and why they should distinguish the new psychology from the spiritualism and psychic research that continued to capture their imaginations (see Coon, 1992; Leary, 1987), or how scientific psychology could coexist harmoniously with religious faith (Pickren, 2000). Nonetheless, awareness and acceptance of the presence of scientific experts in a field where no dividing line between public and expert had formerly been drawn, was growing.

It was into this new 'psychological society' that Burrhus Frederic Skinner (1904–1990) was born, raised, and trained as a psychologist. He developed and communicated his ideas in an era in which both scientific and psychological authority were publicly recognized and accorded special status. His science, and the practices spawned by it, formed a significant part of the body of expert psychological knowledge that was transmitted to American society from the late 1930s until the late 1980s. His struggle to persuade the American public of the value of radical behaviorism as an epistemological and ontological basis, not only for psychology but also for everyday life, provides a magnified, and therefore highly illustrative, picture of psychology's ongoing struggle to be publicly influential as a scientific enterprise. Skinner's attempts to supplant the psychology of everyday experience with his scientifically derived system of behavioral principles also exemplify the discipline's ongoing struggle to gain explanatory ascendance over the subjective experience of everyday life.

In the course of examining Skinner's complex trajectory as a public intellectual, it became clear that a much larger story about the migration of his experimental science from the confines of the operant chamber to real-world application needed to be told. Although Skinner himself achieved popular renown in his own lifetime, many of the now most culturally prominent aspects of his system were developed by scientists and practitioners who extended his work beyond experimental analysis to a wide-ranging technology designed to solve individual and even social problems. No synthetic, contextual, historical account of these developments has been undertaken, despite Skinner's prominence in the history of psychology.[5]

Although Skinner himself served as the lightning rod for public opinion and criticism, hundreds of Skinnerian psychologists, enthralled by the precise science, technological potential, and melioristic underpinnings of Skinner's system, began using the principles of operant psychology, starting in the 1950s, to refashion the human environment and change human behavior.[6] This move from the laboratory to life unfolded most intensely in the ensuing two decades, and continues today. How Skinnerians moved their system beyond the laboratory into the lives of thousands of Americans, the cultural openings and resistances that they encountered, and the effects of this process both on the Skinnerian community itself and the fashioning of the American experience, have not been sufficiently explored.[7]

Thus, a contextual, historical account of the evolution of B.F. Skinner's 'cautious experimental research' from the confines of the operant chamber to the design of total environments for juvenile delinquents, prisoners, and psychiatric patients, to intentional communities and self-help programs, is the subject of this book. I explore this evolution by gradually dismantling the box in which Skinner generated his experimental results – the eponymous Skinner box. I outline how Skinner's experiments with rats and pigeons in small operant chambers inspired experiments with human subjects in an ever-expanding Skinner box until, finally, the box itself disappeared.

One of my major premises in this account is that the most enduring aspect of Skinner's cultural legacy is not his experimental analysis of behavior, his philosophy of radical behaviorism, or his social philosophy – even though many of these contributions propelled his meteoric rise to public prominence in the early 1970s and were subjects of intense popular debate (see Dinsmoor, 1992; Rutherford, 2000, 2003). Instead, I argue that Skinner's most enduring cultural legacy is his *technology* of behavior. Further, I suggest that the acceptance and pervasiveness of this technology was tied to the degree to which it was at least superficially *divorced* from Skinner's philosophy of radical behaviorism[8] and his social philosophy more generally. Some of Skinner's followers realized that despite the widespread appeal of a relatively effective and fairly straightforward set of behavior change techniques, to explicitly link behavior modification to its theoretical and philosophical apparatus often created more headaches than adherents.

Conversely, the ease with which Skinner's experimental principles could be lifted from the laboratory and applied to human problems aligned itself seamlessly with the American technological imperative,[9] or, as historian of psychology William Woodward has put it, with 'the American penchant for making and remaking the environment' (Woodward, 1996, p. 8). In this project, I detail how the technological potential of Skinner's science drove an inexorable process that ultimately resulted in the complete deconstruction of the operant chamber, both literally and figuratively, and propelled the migration of Skinner's principles from the animal laboratory into complex human environments.

I believe the importance of such an account, as a historical project, is self-evident. However, the educated reader may very well ask why we should care about the vestiges of behaviorism. At least superficially, it appears that Skinner's science and technology of behavior have been left behind in the dust of exciting advances in cognitive neuroscience and brain imaging. Like Freud and psychoanalysis, doesn't Skinner seem a bit old-fashioned, behavior modification a bit old school?

Freud and Skinner Are Dead

At the beginning of the twenty-first century, when brain imaging and designer drugs promise ever greater description and control of human behavior by reducing it to its smallest molecular components, some argue that the curtain has been drawn on the psychological divas of the nineteenth and twentieth centuries. These were scientists and theorists, like Freud and Skinner, who extrapolated from individual cases to the very nature of civilization and who confidently inserted their ideas into the popular discourse of their times.[10]

The popular press has repeatedly pronounced Freud and Skinner dead. Many psychological scientists view psychoanalysis and behaviorism as historical curiosities. However, debates about Freud and his putative demise continue to preoccupy the popular imagination. On Monday, 15 May 2000, Freud's status was the subject of a front-page article in the *Los Angeles Times* (see McFarling, 2000). A few years earlier, an article in *Scientific American* tried to convince readers that Freud really wasn't dead (see Horgan, 1996), and on 27 March 2006 an article by Jerry Adler for *Newsweek* magazine proclaimed that Freud was not only *not* dead, he was actually 'in our midst' (see Adler, 2006).

The debate continues. Clearly, Freudian concepts and vocabulary continue to define personal experience and our understanding of the human condition, whether or not we view Freud as a legitimate scientist of the mind. At the institutional level, psychoanalytic societies, meetings, journals, and professionals continue their work, although often operating off the radar screen of the mainstream disciplines of psychiatry and psychology. Woody Allen continues to write and direct, and patients continue to see their analysts. It may be an ironic case of wish fulfillment that Freud is dead only for those who wish him so.

Skinner has also been pronounced dead, which is surely a gross overstatement of the demise of his system both in academic psychology and in everyday life. College professors are fond of repeating a received view of the history of the discipline in which noted linguist Noam Chomsky slayed Skinner with his scathing review of *Verbal Behavior*, Skinner's 1957 book on language (see Chomsky, 1959).[11] As Skinnerian psychologist Carol Pilgrim recently remarked, 'It's not at all difficult to find otherwise sound scholars in psychology who teach their students that behaviorism has gone the way of the dodo bird, most typically at about the time of Chomsky's response (Chomsky, 1959) to Skinner's *Verbal Behavior* (1957)' (in Epting, 2008, p. 51). In this version of events, it is asserted that by the 1960s the bright lights of the cognitive revolution had emancipated psychology from the dark age of behaviorism. More recently, historians have pointed out that this is a grossly oversimplified version of the recent past which, although alluring for pedagogical purposes, fails to suffice as an accurate, or at least sophisticated, analysis of this rather more complex transition (see, for example, Greenwood, 1999, Leahey, 1992; but for the persistence of the notion of a revolution, see Mandler, 2007, especially chapter 10). As Laurence Smith has noted, '[T]he death of behaviorism has been announced with somewhat greater frequency than the actual event has taken place' (Smith, 1992, p. 222; see also Zuriff, 1979).

The major premise of this book is that Skinner, largely through the legacy of his technology of behavior, has had an enduring, although not straightforward, impact on American society. It is the how, when, where, and why of this impact that this volume explores more thoroughly. If Chomsky did not slay Skinner, then where did he go? As we shall see, Skinner seeped out into classrooms, prisons, hospitals, communities, and self-help manuals despite his failure to transform the epistemological basis of psychology or our popular understanding of human nature. I argue that Skinner's system has left its most indelible mark on the American experience, not through his experimental analysis of behavior or his philosophy of radical behaviorism (although academic adherents continue to work productively in both of these areas), but as a result of his technology of behavior. American society continues to be driven by the desire to achieve ever greater control over nature *and* human nature. We continue to view individual behavior as malleable, hold self-improvement as a national creed, and regard social engineering as a desirable enterprise. Skinner's most enduring achievement was to treat human behavior change like any other technological problem. To the extent that we continue to engineer behavior in highly specific ways – and the technology of behavior provides an effective set of engineering tools – Skinner continues to cast a long shadow over the American landscape.

I explore the evolutionary stages of this technology of behavior by expanding and eventually dismantling the box in which Skinner originally generated his experimental results. I outline, using selected case studies, how findings from Skinner's experiments with rats and pigeons in small operant chambers were transformed into a widely employed technology of human behavior over the course of less than two decades. I focus on how the findings and conclusions drawn from this basic work came to be applied to human populations and problems starting in the late 1950s, and then began to flourish throughout the 1960s and 1970s. I do not, however, attempt a synoptic or comprehensive account of these applications. Their sheer volume would necessitate a historical handbook which could easily run to many hundreds of pages. Instead, I have chosen projects that were considered pioneering or attracted significant attention in the professional or popular literature, such as Harold Cohen's CASE project for juvenile delinquents (see chapter 4) and Teodoro Ayllon and Nathan Azrin's token economy for schizophrenics at Anna State Hospital (see chapter 3).

One of the themes that emerges from my account is that in venturing beyond the box, Skinnerian psychologists encountered both cultural openings and cultural resistances that deeply influenced the development and impact of their technology of behavior. Cultural openings provided Skinnerian psychologists with opportunities to transport their techniques beyond the confines of the laboratory and prove their usefulness to society at large. However, the leap from the laboratory to life was not boundless. Technologists of behavior soon found that with these opportunities came resistances towards, and sometimes restrictions placed upon, their work. In some cases these resistances led to organized attacks, as in the case of legal action and federal regulations in response to some of the prison programs I describe in chapter 4. At other times resistance was expressed through attacks on Skinner's own character, as I detail in chapter 1. In order to understand the impact of these openings and resistances on the science and technology of behavior and its social influence, I weave both intra-disciplinary and extra-disciplinary factors into my account and oscillate intentionally between the scientific and professional world of the Skinnerian psychologist and the social and political context of the United States from the 1950s to the 1970s. Only by moving beyond the artificiality of the internalist/externalist divide can we trace the significance of Skinner's technology of behavior in American life.

Given these aims, I should outline certain caveats. In writing *Beyond the Box*, my aim is not to promote a Skinner revival, although others have been tempted to do so (see Barash, 2005, for a recent exposition on why Skinner's emphasis on a rigorously objective study of behavior and rejection of free will should be resurrected). Nor is my aim to argue that cognitivism is actually behaviorism in a new form (see Leahey, 1992, p. 316, and Leahey, 2001, pp. 305–6 for a version of this argument). I do not propose that we are all behaviorists, whether we realize it or not (see Roediger, 2004, for a version of this claim). Rather, my intention is to explore when, where, and how Skinnerian ideas and approaches have proved useful, although not uncontroversial, by tracing the evolution of behavior analysis from a basic experimental science, heavily reliant on the highly controlled conditions of the operant chamber, to a successful technology of human behavior that has taken hold in a number of significant cultural milieus. In the process, I hope to elucidate a number of historiographic and macro-historical issues using aspects of Skinner's science and technology as illustrative, interesting, and substantive examples.

Historiographic Issues

Devoting a whole book to Skinner's technology of behavior conveys the implicit belief that there remains something important to say about B.F. Skinner's behaviorism, both for psychology and for life more generally. As I alluded to above, this is not an uncontroversial position; many psychologists have resoundingly dismissed his system, characterizing it as naïve, misguided, and theoretically bankrupt. John A. Mills concludes his analysis of the fate of behaviorism generally, including Skinner's technology of behavior, by linking its initial success and ultimate demise with the rise and fall of modernism, noting that by the late twentieth century, the 'sun of modernism, which nourished behaviorism ..., has sunk beneath the horizon. Bereft of its support, the psychological technologies of yesteryear are pale, limp, and etiolated' (Mills, 1998, p. 193).

However, to state that Skinner's behaviorism, and especially his technology of behavior, has faded completely away is almost as tenuous a historical claim as stating that modernism has fallen, and does not do justice to the myriad and intricate ways in which any far-reaching school of thought, such as behaviorism, psychoanalysis, or even modernism, leaves its mark on the culture it has inhabited. In this book, I challenge the claim that the sun has set on Skinner's technology of behavior by reconstructing the stories of those followers and students who spread Skinnerian science and technology into the cracks and crevices of academic, applied, and popular psychology from the mid-1950s through the 1970s. I argue that the sum of this work, more so than its individual parts, has left indelible traces on the way Americans conceptualize themselves and their experiences even into the early twenty-first century.

Although there is a rich literature on the psychologization of the self and the making of a psychological society in twentieth-century America,[12] most of these accounts have focused on the role of psychoanalytic, humanistic, and even cognitive theories, or on the role of testing and psychotherapy, in accomplishing this psychologization. Little attention has been paid to how Skinner's system may have shaped the psychological self, perhaps because it has seemed ridiculously incongruous to do so. After all, as Martin and Barresi (2006) have recently noted, 'In general, introspectionists and behaviorists had little to say about the self, and nothing to say about it of lasting importance' (p. 245). However, if one can step outside the strictures of Skinner's philosophical position, which did indeed deny individual agency and cast the self in an almost unrecognizable form, and instead examine the resonances and disjunctures of a technology of behavior within the culture that both gave rise to and received it, it becomes much more difficult to discount his influence and vanquish the technology of behavior from the historical literature on the making of a psychological society.

In most standard textbooks on the history of psychology, accounts of Skinner's technology of behavior have suffered a strange, truncated fate. Although most standard accounts include a generous section or chapter on Skinner and his science of behavior, and may even mention his controversial books *Beyond Freedom and Dignity* and *Walden Two*, they rarely delve into the development of the technology of behavior. This is due in large part to the aforementioned storyline about the demise of behaviorism and the rise of cognitivism, coupled with the tendency of disciplinary histories to focus on classic experiments, great people, and grand theories rather than application. Be that as it may, this oversight may be excusable on other grounds entirely. Even from a strict disciplinary standpoint, it is generally true that Skinnerian scientists and practitioners have both intentionally and unintentionally removed themselves from mainstream psychology, in effect writing themselves out of – or at least making themselves less visible to – those who survey the history of the field. The reasons for and effects of this institutional marginalization will be explored throughout the book, but I will focus specifically on this issue in the concluding chapter.

This truncation may also be due to the fact that in developing a technology of behavior, Skinnerian psychologists have, in effect, created a product that has been relatively easy to give away, both to consumers and to other practitioners. As a result, the development of this technology has at times taken place outside psychology, sometimes even without psychologists, and hence its impact may be understated in disciplinary accounts and is largely absent from the internalist stories psychologists often tell each other and their students.

In many of the historical developments I recount, the intricacies of the public's relationship with Skinner's technology of behavior provide a strong subtext, or sometimes even the main storyline. In unraveling these intricacies, I intentionally stray from strict and precise disciplinary definitions of behaviorism, behavior analysis, and behavior modification. This is entirely necessary because the lay consumers of Skinner's technology of behavior did not use these terms in the same way formally trained practitioners did. I intentionally fluctuate between accounts of internal disciplinary developments and their external reception and appropriation to highlight the permeability of these two cultures.

Historians of psychology are just beginning to relax the tightness of their grip on strict disciplinary histories that generally ignore the ways in which the terms, phenomena, procedures, and products of the laboratory both arise from and return to the lay culture of which they are, ultimately, a part.[13] Kroker (2003), in his 'anti-disciplinarian analysis' of introspection, makes the point – and it bears repeating – that the stories psychologists and other scientists tell one another almost always focus on scientific, technical, and professional developments deemed internal to their fields, and rarely relate how these developments are appropriated and transformed outside of them.

What scientists tell each other aside, there is now a large body of work by historians and sociologists of science exploring how 'laboratory-made knowledge ... emerges into the world outside' (Golinski, 2005, p. 92). This work includes analyses of how the culture of the laboratory itself shapes the production of knowledge and how this knowledge subsequently makes its way from the laboratory into society (e.g., Latour, 1987; Latour and Woolgar, 1986; Shapin and Schaffer, 1985; Whitley, 1985).[14] Some scholars have proposed that the successful exportation of scientific knowledge involves certain characteristic processes in which scientific facts are decontextualized from the unavoidably local sites where they were created, and are subsequently rendered more dramatic and forceful. For example, the presentation of scientific results to non-specialist audiences involves the removal of both the intellectual and social contexts in which the results were generated, as well as the contingencies and limits of generalizability that govern their truth status. This often serves to inflate the status and certainty of scientific results. Thus, to make successful claims to universality, the place of provenance of such facts has to be either hidden, or the laboratory has to be elevated to a generic 'truth spot,' as Gieryn (2002) has shown.

Other scholars have argued that this process involves not 'generalization to universal laws instantiable elsewhere' (Rouse, 1987, p. 125), but the successive and systematic reproduction of the material and cultural conditions prevailing in the original site of knowledge production in other settings. In my account of how Skinner's system moved from the laboratory to life, I explore how both of these processes operated, and propose that the proliferation of the technology of behavior depended, perhaps paradoxically, *both* on asserting its claims to universal effectiveness *and* on physically reproducing or discursively re-invoking the materials and culture of the laboratory and the trope of a technological approach to human behavior, across multiple settings.

Another fundamental premise underlying this analysis of Skinner's legacy beyond the box is that scientific terminology, and *psychological* scientific terminology in particular, has the potential, when introduced into the popular lexicon, to exert a lasting and widespread effect on how we experience ourselves. As one historian of psychology has remarked, '[C]hanges in psychological language signify psychological change in their own right' (Richards, 1996, p. 6). Some historians and philosophers of psychology believe that ways of labeling and talking about experience actually circulate back to shape the nature of the experience itself (e.g., Hacking, 1995). Taken to its extreme, this argument could end up with language actually *creating* experience, where no corresponding experience existed before.

In this work, I subscribe to a milder version of this claim. In the case of Skinner, I believe that his use of a specialized language to describe the findings from his experimental analysis of behavior was his attempt to characterize observed phenomena, and to lay claim to a body of specialized knowledge. But in creating this specialized language and using it to describe human behavior, Skinner introduced a vocabulary that both changed and challenged how people conceptualized themselves and others in some rather dramatic ways. Thus, to paraphrase Richards (1996), nobody had their behavior modified in quite the same way before the term 'behavior modification' came to be used to describe that experience. Reinforcements and rewards took on different connotations in a post-Skinnerian world, and our relationship to them changed. But rather than digress further on this point, I will take it up more explicitly in chapter 5 when I explore Skinnerian principles in self-help.

Moving beyond the Box

Skinner is the foundational figure around which my account develops, but he is not the main subject of this book.[15] I devote the first chapter to his role as a public intellectual, but I do not delve extensively into the underpinnings of his science or his philosophy. For information about his experimental work, the reader can go directly to the source and consult Skinner's foundational work *The Behavior of Organisms* (Skinner, 1938) and his subsequent book with Charles Ferster, *Schedules of Reinforcement* (Ferster and Skinner, 1957). Almost any introductory psychology or learning theory textbook will offer the basics of operant conditioning. Suffice it to say that a cornerstone of operant psychology is the observation and demonstration that behavior can be controlled by its consequences, and that the manipulation of these consequences can produce precise and replicable behavioral effects (for an overview of B.F. Skinner's behaviorism in twelve fundamental points, see Delprato and Midgley, 1992). For his philosophy of radical behaviorism, the interested reader would be well advised to consult reputable secondary sources (e.g., Coleman, 1984, 1991; Day, 1983; Day and Moore, 1995; Moore, 2008; Morris, 1993; Rutherford, 2005; Zuriff, 1980, 1985). It is an unfortunate but well-known fact that most psychologists continue to misunderstand and misrepresent Skinner's philosophy, especially its relationship with other forms of behaviorism.[16] In fact, there is a small cottage industry concerning misrepresentations of Skinner and his system, especially as it occurs in textbook accounts (see DeBell and Harless, 1992; Hobbs, Cornwell, and Chiesa, 2000; Todd and Morris, 1983; Wyatt, 1993).

The main subjects of my account are the psychologists, scientists, and practitioners who extended Skinner's principles to the measurement and manipulation of *human* behavior in experimental, institutional, and eventually naturalistic settings. The titular use of the phrase 'beyond the box' is meaningful on several levels; I employ it both metaphorically and literally. First, Skinner conducted the bulk of his experimental analyses within the confines of an operant chamber that he designed to run his experimental subjects – mainly pigeons and rats. Much to his chagrin, this apparatus came to be known as the Skinner box, and remains a key feature of the operant laboratory to this day.

In its early incarnations, the Skinner box consisted of several components. It contained an operandum, which for the rat was a lever that could be pressed, and for the pigeon a disk that could be pecked. When the animal emitted the operant – the lever press or disk peck – a chute would deliver a pellet of food. The food delivery could be automatically programmed to occur on specific reinforcement schedules, say one pellet after every third lever press, or one pellet for the first response after thirty seconds. Skinner also designed a device for automatically recording the animals' operant response rates. Each operant chamber was equipped with a cumulative recorder that recorded rates of response, generating elegant graphs for subsequent inspection by the researcher. In more elaborate experiments, food reinforcement could be programmed to occur not only on specific schedules, but also variably in the presence of certain lights or sounds. Lattal (2004) offers an informative history of the cumulative recorder from the 1930s to the present, including photographs. He writes: 'The cumulative recorder was to early behavior analysts what the microscope was to early biologists' (Lattal, 2004, p. 329). That is, it allowed them to see patterns and lawfulness in behavior that could not be discerned through casual observation.

Ultimately, Skinner showed with this work that response rates could be determined reliably and precisely by the schedule of reinforcement used to generate them. He showed that animal behavior could be precisely controlled by its consequences. His magnum opus in this area was the book *Schedules of Reinforcement* written with his colleague Charles Ferster, published in 1957. Although Skinner never directly conducted experiments with humans, based on this work he did not consider it a huge leap to assume that human behavior could be precisely controlled by its consequences as well. He left it to others to explore and demonstrate exactly whether, and how, this would work. These demonstrations are the subject of much of this account. As it turns out, at issue was not so much the question of *whether* they would work (most Skinnerians held an unwavering faith in the efficacy of their techniques), but *how* a technology of behavior would fare in the world outside the laboratory and how this exportation would in turn influence the forms the technology took.

After a discussion of Skinner's status as a public intellectual in the first chapter, in chapter 2 I describe the work of three Skinnerian psychologists who physically expanded the operant chamber in order to study human behavior: Charles Ferster, Ogden Lindsley, and Sidney Bijou. To accommodate their human subjects, they designed and constructed human-sized or room-sized Skinner boxes. Although this work was purely experimental in nature, I explore its relation to early efforts at application that were already unfolding in the Skinnerian community. In chapters 3 and 4, I show how the human Skinner box was re-envisioned and expanded to accommodate larger-scale behavior change projects taking the form of programs in total institutions such as psychiatric hospitals (chapter 3) and prisons (chapter 4). In these settings, applied behavior analysts no longer worked with subjects confined to boxes or even rooms, but the patients and prisoners involved in their programs were nonetheless physically confined to settings, such as hospital wards or prison cellblocks, that allowed for a high degree of behavioral control. Additionally, the emphasis on measurement and control was maintained, but intervention and behavior change were the ultimate pragmatic objectives.

In chapter 5, I dismantle the box completely. I show how, in the 1970s, Skinnerian psychologists wrote self-help manuals in which they applied basic behavioral principles to everyday problems such as how to lose weight, give up smoking, or become more assertive. Although the readers of these self-improvement manuals lacked the luxury of a precisely controllable environment, they were instructed to harness the power of the environmental contingencies they could set up themselves. They were exhorted to abandon recourse to willpower and adopt the rhetoric of self-control. I show how many of the principles presented in Skinnerian self-help and self-improvement manuals have seeped imperceptibly into the social and cultural milieu we now inhabit and how the authors of these texts accomplished this sleight of hand.

Finally, in chapter 6, life as laboratory becomes community as laboratory. Here I describe how Skinnerian principles were taken up by devotees of Skinner's fictional utopian novel, *Walden Two*, in the late 1960s and early 1970s as the basis for engineering entire communities. In this period, groups of *Walden Two*–inspired communitarians attempted to translate Skinner's ideas into a version of the good life in real life. In this chapter, I examine two of these communities in detail, Twin Oaks and Los Horcones, and discuss how these attempts to bring the laboratory to community actually played out.

Thus, the phrase 'beyond the box' is employed to evoke a variety of analytic possibilities. I employ it to argue that the physical design and construction of the operant chamber was a highly significant locus for research and application in the Skinnerian tradition and exerted a powerful – perhaps even constitutive – influence on the development of a technology of human behavior, a point to which I will return in my conclusion. The gradual physical expansion, and finally complete deconstruction, of the box itself from a small chamber, to a room, to a building, to a community, to a rhetoric for self-improvement, also provides a convenient trope for structuring my account. More importantly, it facilitates an analysis of how this laboratory-made knowledge emerged into the world outside. The transfer of the phenomena of the operant laboratory to sites beyond their point of origin involved a variety of different professional, scientific, and rhetorical manoeuvres. These included moving from the basic to the applied (although this distinction was often blurred), from the local to the universal, from the specific to the general, from the private to the public, and from the academic to the popular. As Golinski (2005) has noted, 'The local setting where scientific knowledge originates is crucial, but the wider realm beyond its walls can also be viewed as an arena in which knowledge is constructed' (p. 37).

Finally, the phrase is also a play on the title of Skinner's best-known book, *Beyond Freedom and Dignity*. In this work, Skinner called on his readers to see beyond freedom to the enormous potential of a world more intentionally controlled and engineered. This plea evoked intense and widespread criticism, and inspired attacks upon both his personal integrity and his professional work. In reading the account that follows, I call on readers to see beyond the box to the spirit of social meliorism that, despite some missteps along the way, motivated many technologists of behavior as they transported Skinner from the laboratory to life.

chapter 1

A Visible Scientist:
B.F. Skinner as Public Intellectual

For perhaps the first time in American history, a professor of psychology has acquired the celebrity of a movie or TV star.

Hall, 1972, p. 68

To try to reimagine the celebrity status B.F. Skinner enjoyed in the 1970s, dislodge the image of a white-coated laboratory scientist patiently teaching pigeons to peck for grain. Instead, imagine Skinner as one of *Esquire*'s '100 Most Important People' in 1970 and the subject of a *Time* magazine cover story in 1971. Imagine Skinner as the prominent Harvard academic who withdrew from bench science by the early 1960s[1] to develop and promulgate a controversial social philosophy, culminating in the publication of a *New York Times* best-selling book. Imagine Skinner bringing his message to the talk-show circuit with appearances on *Phil Donahue*, *Firing Line*, and the *Dick Cavett Show* (Bjork, 1993; Knapp, 1996; Skinner, 1983a). Imagine, if you can, that 'talk of Skinner was stirred into cocktail conversation' (Hilts, 1973a, p. 18).

It may be somewhat easier to appreciate the extent of Skinner's influence in the field of psychology itself. In surveys of disciplinary eminence, Skinner's name always rises to the top of the list (Haggbloom et al., 2002; Korn, Davis, and Davis, 1991). Over a career that spanned more than sixty years, he published over twenty books. He extended his science of behavior to the design of cultures (Skinner, 1961a) and to the amelioration of social practices (Skinner, 1953, 1971a). Skinner's science of behavior became the foundation for the contemporary discipline of behavior analysis, whose professional organization, the Association for Behavior Analysis International, currently has over 5,000 members in the United States, and 13,000 members in affiliated chapters in the United States and around the world (Twyman, 2007). Numerous behavior analytic journals, such as *Behavior Analyst, Journal of the Experimental Analysis of Behavior, Journal of Applied Behavior Analysis, Analysis of Verbal Behavior, Behavior and Social Issues,* and the *European Journal of Behavior Analysis, Behavior and Philosophy* – among others – carry on the Skinnerian tradition. You can even become a certified Skinnerian – a Board-Certified Behavior Analyst, or BCBA (see http://www.bacb.com/).

For all of these reasons, Skinner is a notable figure in the history of psychology. But it is clear that Skinner's historical significance transcends simple disciplinary eminence. To use the metaphor from the title, his significance extends 'beyond the box.' He is an important figure in the history of twentieth-century American intellectual life.

By the late 1960s, if not earlier, Skinner had become, in the words of communications researcher Rae Goodell, a 'visible scientist' (Goodell, 1977).[2] According to Goodell, like other visible scientists Skinner circumvented traditional channels of scientific communication and sent his message straight to the public. By 1990, Skinner's utopian novel *Walden Two* had sold over 2.5 million copies (Bjork, 1993, p. 162). His 1971 book, *Beyond Freedom and Dignity* (*BFD*, Skinner, 1971a), was on the *New York Times* best-seller list for a total of twenty-six weeks. Skinner reported that, after *BFD*, people would approach him at restaurants and other public venues to inquire if he were 'Professor Skinner,' having seen him on television. In one instance, a young admirer identified Skinner and turned to her friends, exclaiming, 'Now you have met a celebrity!' (Skinner, 1983a, p. 319). Evidently, Skinner and his publisher were quite surprised by the popularity of the book. As Skinner's daughter Julie Vargas noted, '[T]hey certainly did not expect it to be a best-seller and printed far too few. And that was a very big surprise, both to him and to the publisher, when it was a best-seller, because none of his other books had been' (Vargas, 2000, interview with author).

As a public intellectual, Skinner was noteworthy in at least three respects. First, the content of his message and his vision for society at times resonated, and at other times collided, with several prominent strains of American social thought (Bjork, 1996; Smith, 1996b; Rutherford, 2003). In some cases, he received popular attention because he provided novel and sensational solutions to age-old problems such as how to bring up baby, how to teach Johnny, and how to live the 'good life.' In other cases, he sparked the ire of popular audiences because his views subverted traditional American values such as the right to self-determination and belief in free will. In this chapter, I introduce Skinner as a public intellectual and the incursion of Skinnerian themes into popular culture by presenting three of the projects that lured him away from the laboratory and earned him recognition beyond the ivory tower. I also show how these projects were received by the American public, and argue that popular portrayals of Skinner's work were complexly intertwined with the political and socio-cultural trends of post–Second World War America.

Skinner was also notable because, unlike Freud, Rogers, Maslow, or Dr Phil, he embodied the psychologist as bench scientist to a greater extent than possibly any other psychologist of his renown in the history of the discipline. His system was built upon findings from animal-based laboratory work executed with the highest degree of experimental control. His scientific philosophy emphasized observation, measurement, and induction, and he prided himself on being data-driven rather than theory-driven. Theory, in Skinner's view, was useful only if it remained as close to the data as possible, ideally serving as a parsimonious summary of a large set of empirical results (see Skinner, 1950).

The particular challenges and problems that this created for Skinner's public image were considerable. In many ways, Skinner's embodiment of the positivist, scientific ideal in psychology created serious apprehension in audiences whose expectations about the science of mental life were appreciably different from their expectations about natural science. Rogers, Maslow, and Freud, although each controversial in his own way, were not stereotyped as white-coated, rat-running laboratory scientists, and thus did not suffer quite the same fate as Skinner in the popular imagination.[3] I explore this contention later in this chapter, and propose that portrayals of Skinner, not only as a scientist and a psychologist, but as a human being, were conflated with attitudes towards his theory and towards the relevance of *scientific* psychology for self-understanding more generally (see also Rutherford, 2000).

Finally, Skinner was ardently committed to the application of his ideas through a technology of behavior. In fact, he viewed technology as the preeminent concern of all scientific activity (Smith, 1992, 1996a). As a result, he often inverted the traditional relationship between theory and application by applying first, and theorizing later. Throughout his life and career, he wanted to change the world in which he lived by applying the principles of operant psychology in a scheme of potentially widespread social and behavioral engineering. In this way, Skinner was truly a product of American culture. As Woodward (1996) has noted of Skinner's writing, 'As works consciously constructed during a period of technological optimism in

American life, Skinner's writings convey a peculiarly "hands on" social philosophy. They extend to the social and personal realms a philosophy of technology that ... has long been ingrained in the American penchant for making and remaking the environment' (p. 8). As a behavioral engineer, Skinner breached the sacrosanct divide between basic science and application. This breach, although controversial, earned him an audience outside the ivory tower: 'Fred Skinner's excursions into technology may have offended the sensibilities of his fellow scientists, but they have also brought him a popularity – or infamy, depending on your point of view – that few scientists ever achieve' (Rice, 1968, p. 95).

Skinner's zeal to remake the environment was matched only by the zeal of his followers. Students, colleagues, and devotees of the Skinnerian world view took Skinner's principles and ideas and applied them in the real world to a host of individual, community, and social problems. As practitioners of applied behavior analysis (as the applied branch of Skinner's system became known), these psychologists were among the most effective behavioral engineers of the mid-twentieth century. The rest of this book is about some of their efforts to take Skinner's system beyond the box. Before we get to their stories, however, let us see how Skinner himself moved from the laboratory to life.

The Laboratory of Life

Baby in a Box

Although it was not until the early 1970s that Skinner reached the height of his popular renown, very early in his career he was interested not only in remaking the environment, but also in presenting his ideas to an audience beyond academia. His first article for the popular press, written as the Second World War was coming to a close, featured a device that he had invented to solve a domestic, rather than a scientific, problem.[4] Skinner and his wife, Eve, were expecting their second child. Although excited about another addition to the family, Eve was not looking forward to the increase in menial physical labor that would accompany raising a second child. Could Skinner the scientist and father come up with a better way to bring up baby?

An inveterate gadgeteer, Skinner once remarked to a group of friends: 'There has never been a problem that I didn't try and solve with a gadget' (Skinner, 1971c). So in response to his wife's concerns, Skinner designed and built an enclosed, temperature- and humidity-controlled crib with a

Plexiglas front and a stretched canvas bed. He called his invention the baby tender, but later renamed it the air crib. His intention was to help make child care easier and more efficient, and to provide a more comfortable environment for the baby.[5] This was accomplished in a variety of ways, which Skinner outlined to the readers of *Ladies Home Journal* in an article entitled 'Baby Care Can Be Modernized.' The editors decided on a somewhat punchier title, however, and the article appeared instead as 'Baby in a Box – Introducing the Mechanical Baby Tender' (Skinner, 1945). Unfortunately but inevitably, the crib almost immediately became known as the Skinner baby box.

In his article, Skinner extolled the virtues of the air crib for both parents and babies alike. Because the temperature and humidity were controlled inside the crib, a baby could wear only a diaper and had no need of blankets. Mothers would be relieved of some laundry, and children would be less likely to become tangled in their bedclothes and were freer to move about. The environment inside the air crib was also quieter and more germ-free than a regular crib. Babies slept better, had fewer rashes, and developed better musculature. Although not sound-proofed (Skinner reassured parents that they would be able to hear their child's cries), the air crib nonetheless provided a more controlled environment than that provided by a regular crib. The level of control was actually quite precise, as demonstrated in this excerpt from an article in the *Industrial Bulletin of Arthur D. Little Inc*:

> Dr. Skinner has used the crib throughout the life of his daughter, now 16-months old, and reports that she has benefited from the experience. Even in small houses or apartments, the crib is said to enable the baby to devise its own routine around the feeding or bathing schedule. In one instance when the Skinner baby was changed from 4 to 3 meals a day, she began to wake up an hour before breakfast time. By raising the temperature in the air crib, thus helping her retain the warmth from her evening meal, her waking was postponed for the necessary hour.[6]

Reactions to the air crib were mixed. As Skinner himself had noted, the editors' use of the title 'Baby in a Box' probably did little to help the image of the baby tender. In the second volume of his autobiography, he reported an observation made by one of his colleagues: 'The only time that human beings are subject to boxes is when they are dead' (Skinner, 1979, p. 305). He also noted the inescapable similarity between the baby box and the 'Skinner box,' an experimental chamber used to test operant principles with animals (notably, however, Skinner never conducted experiments with the air crib).

Despite these unfortunate allusions, responses generally fell into one of two categories. In the first category were those who indeed thought that the air crib was at best a crazy contraption invented by a hare-brained scientist, and at worst a dangerous device in which the baby would suffer emotional and physical harm. According to these critics, raising children in boxes was a sign of parental neglect, and would result in permanent damage to the child's psyche. In the second category, were those who saw the baby box as a welcome addition to the growing array of household technologies that promised to streamline domestic tasks and make parenting easier. These reactions tended to highlight both the labor-saving aspects of the air crib and its potential for producing healthier, happier, and even smarter children.[7] While those in the first camp decried the mechanization of mothering, those in the latter perceived it as a sign of technological and social progress.

To what extra-individual factors can we attribute these two divergent sets of reactions? I would argue that several features specific to the socio-cultural landscape of the immediate post–Second World War era can help make sense of these polarized views (see also Rutherford, 2003). First, to help us understand the positive reception of the air crib, it is important to remember that as the Second World War drew to a close and the 1950s began, the United States was deep in the throes of a better-living campaign. After the paucity of luxury goods during the war years, better living in the 1950s meant increased material consumption. Specifically, this increased consumption focused on the acquisition of household appliances that would bring the suburban housewife into the world of the future.[8] Skinner was not unaware of this trend, writing in his *Ladies Home Journal* article, 'It is quite in the spirit of the "world of the future" to make favorable conditions available everywhere through simple mechanical means' (Skinner, 1945, p. 136).

The decade following the conclusion of the war was a period of both economic prosperity and techno-fervor. The invention of new appliances, and the increased production of appliances that had not been manufactured during the war, meant that Americans were bringing home new washing machines, vacuum cleaners, and television sets – why not a new and improved crib? Many of these devices promised increased control and mastery over the domestic environment. Like other new appliances, in addition to saving labor, the baby tender also offered a technological improvement over traditional practices. While vacuum cleaners and washing machines promised cleaner floors and whiter clothes, the baby tender promised smarter and healthier babies. For example, a 1947 *Life* article 'Boxes for Babies' featured John Gray, Jr, alert and content in his tender, with the caption 'John Gray Jr. plays happily in his box. Like Debby Skinner he has never had a cold or a stomach upset, is smarter than the average child' (p. 73). In 'Box-Reared Babies,' a 1954 *Time* magazine article, readers learned of Roy and Ray Hope, a pair of six-year-old 'bright-eyed twins' who had spent 'the first 18 months of their lives in a Skinner baby box.' These 'disarmingly normal' young boys were featured as pictures of physical and psychological health. The mother of the twins expressed her enthusiasm about the device, reporting that 'the box is a boon to mothers because it cuts down on laundry and bathing' ('Box-Reared Babies,' 1954, p. 66).

But despite this receptivity to household technology, there were still vehement objections to the air crib. One primary objection was that using an enclosed crib would weaken the emotional bonds between parents and babies, leading to later maladjustment – maybe even delinquency. In 1946, Dr Benjamin Spock published his *Common Sense Book of Baby and Child Care*, in which – in direct contrast to the Watsonian, behaviorist approach – he urged parents to be more affectionate, more natural, and more responsive towards their children. The image of box-reared babies appeared incongruent with this more nurturant approach, despite Skinner's point that parents would use the air crib in the same way as a traditional crib, that is, only when the child was put down to sleep.

The 1950s also witnessed the apogee of psychoanalytic influence on popular culture (Buhle, 1998; Hale, 1995). Psychoanalytic concepts and ideas infused popular writing, theater, television, and cinema (Gabbard and Gabbard, 1999; Walker, 1993). Psychodynamic theory emphasized the importance of very early infancy and infant attachment on subsequent development, and especially the appropriate care and ministrations of the mother. The importance of healthy, early mothering became widely accepted and undoubtedly exacerbated cultural anxiety about the baby tender.

Indeed, the shifting roles of the mother and the housewife preoccupied the national psyche. In the 1950s, women were often faced with contradictory messages and social expectations. As historian Lynn Spigel has explained, 'Although middle and working-class women had been encouraged by popular media to enter traditionally male occupations during the war, they were now told to return to their homes where they could have babies and make color-coordinated meals' (Spigel, 1992, p. 41). As thousands of middle- and upper-middle-class women struggled with their forced retreat, valium, dubbed 'mother's little helper,' both provided personal relief from existential angst and conveniently subdued the wanderlust that threatened happy homes and happy husbands. As Jonathan Metzl has written, '[P]sychopharmaceuticals came of age in a postwar consumer culture intimately concerned with the role of mothers in maintaining individual and communal peace of mind' (Metzl, 2003, p. 72).

Some of the reactions to the baby tender reflected this reversion to ultra-traditional sex-role stereotypes. Was the mother of a box-raised child shirking her primary role as maternal caregiver? As one anonymous 'Reader of the Times' wrote of the tender, 'It is the most ridiculous, crazy invention ever heard of. Caging this baby up like an animal, just to relieve the Mother of a little more work.'[9] Another reader wrote to Skinner accusingly, 'Think of the wives of soldiers and sailors – they have children to take care of, sometimes their husbands are dead – do they put their baby in a contraption – No! They give their babys [sic] the love and affection they need.'[10] In one article, the father of a box-reared baby reaffirmed sex-role stereotypes by remarking, 'People, particularly women, shy away from such unglamorous devices ... They prefer the conventional crib, with all its frills and ribbons'[11]

So while being a good *housewife* in 1950s America meant participating in the consumer culture by purchasing appliances, tranquillizers, and time on the psychoanalytic couch, being a good *mother* meant resisting the robot nurse, embracing the bassinet, and devoting oneself full-time to bringing up baby. Although Skinner could not have anticipated how his invention would enter into these national debates, by circulating his ideas in the popular press and entering the public arena both as a scientist and as a father, he exposed himself to both praise and censure. With his 1945 *Ladies Home Journal* article, he set himself on a path towards public intellectual that would take just over twenty more years to come to full fruition. In the meantime, there was another problem to be solved with the help of technology.

Teaching by Machine

Skinner's second daughter, Deborah, whose arrival had provided the impetus for the air crib, also provided the inspiration for Skinner's next invention, albeit indirectly. While visiting Deborah's math class during Parents' Day at Shady Hill School, Skinner became convinced that traditional teaching methods required serious revision. In observing Deborah's teacher, he realized that, in a typical classroom of twenty to thirty students, a teacher could not possibly reinforce correct answers immediately, and could not tailor the learning process so that each student proceeded at his or her own pace. Some students sat idly while others struggled to keep up. His engineering spirit kicked in once again, and he spent a large part of the next seven or eight years working, writing, and collaborating on a solution to this problem: programmed instruction.

Over the course of the 1950s and 1960s, Skinner published numerous articles on teaching machines and programmed instruction (e.g., Skinner, 1954, 1958, 1961b). Unlike his approach to the air crib, however, his first impulse was not to publish in the popular press. Whereas in the case of the air crib, his daughter Julie remarked, 'He probably wrote the article because he had invented this neat gadget and thought the public ought to have the advantage of it' (Vargas, 2000, interview with author), in the case of teaching machines, Skinner was concerned with applying experimental principles rigorously to the learning process. He also knew that he would not have to advertise the invention; there was plenty of interest from industry.

Programmed instruction was an approach in which students were exposed to course material in small incremental steps via frames presented in a box-like apparatus. They were required to generate a response to a question about the material, and could then immediately compare their response to the right answer. The presentation of the material was finely tuned to ensure very few mistakes, on the principle that getting the right answer – right away – was maximally reinforcing. Presenting the material in frames also prevented cheating; students could not uncover the right answer without first providing their own, and all of their incorrect responses could be recorded and used as data in revising and improving the programs.[12]

Although Skinner was never completely successful in commercially marketing and mass-producing the air crib,[13] the teaching machine was of great interest to the educational technology industry. However, articles about the machines in the popular press expressed divided opinions about the robot teacher. In a pattern similar to the air crib responses, reactions generally fell into two categories. The first category included reactions from parents, teachers, and journalists who saw it as a dehumanizing force, a threat to the development of the teacher-student bond that was seen as an essential element of education in the liberal-humanistic tradition. In the second category were positive and enthusiastic responses from those who saw the teaching machine as a technological solution to improving education so that American students could keep up with their Cold War competitors in the marketplace of ideas. Again, Skinner's own intentions for the device were largely overlooked. Just as he did not intend the air crib to replace mothers, he did not intend the teaching machines to replace teachers. He argued that with more time freed up from the rote task of presenting material, teachers could spend more time in individualized instruction.[14] Despite this, the threat of technological unemployment also fuelled critics' anxiety.

The teaching machine quickly became one of the focal points of the educational technology movement that received its fullest expression in the early-to-mid 1960s (see, for example, Boroff, 1963; Cuban, 1986; 'What's Happening in Education?' 1967). Starting in the 1950s, film, television, and other audiovisual devices infiltrated classrooms across the country. In 1953, the first educational television network was established (Packer, 1963), and a decade later there were sixty-two educational television stations serving the students of the United States (Boroff, 1963). One of the major sources of money for the educational technology movement was the Ford Fund for the Advancement of Education (Seligman, 1958). The Ford Fund poured millions of dollars into the education industry in this period, responding in part to a perceived teacher shortage, and in part to the need to improve educational practices for students across widely ranging ability levels. In addition, there was national concern that American students were falling behind their Communist peers and that the United States, without superior intellectual stock, would lose the space race, the arms race, and ultimately its position of global political supremacy. The Cold War loomed large.

A number of articles in the mid-1950s announced Skinner's work with the machines (see, for example, 'Mechanical Teacher,' 1954; 'Miracle Gadget,' 1954; 'Teaching by Machine,' 1954; Ubell, 1954). These articles appeared after Skinner's first public demonstration of a machine for teaching spelling and arithmetic at a conference entitled 'Current Trends in Psychology' at the University of Pittsburgh in the spring of 1954 (Skinner, 1954). By the early 1960s, Skinner's teaching machines and programmed instruction were proclaimed by some to be the most radical of the new educational technologies. It was anticipated that the machines and the programs fed into them would completely change the face of education. *Time* magazine reported that programmed learning 'promises the first real innovation in teaching since the invention of movable type in the fifteenth century ... Conceivably, programing might change school design and the entire social structure of U.S. youth' ('Programed Learning,' 1961, p. 36). *Fortune* magazine similarly enthused that programmed instruction 'could, in the next decade or two revolutionize education ...' (Boehm, 1960, p. 176). And in *Science Digest*: 'A few months ago, thousands of school children from coast to coast were quietly subjected to what may turn out to be the greatest educational revolution in history. They began the first large-scale experiment in learning, not from human teachers, but from teaching machines' (Gilmore, 1961, p. 77).

Obviously, there was widespread hope that the implementation of programmed instruction would greatly improve education at the elementary, secondary, and post-secondary levels. This hope extended to other forms of educational technology as well. But while many were enthusiastic and optimistic about teaching machines, the next 'revolution in education' was not embraced by all – especially as the consumer culture of the 1950s gave way to the counterculture of the 1960s.

As the sixties unfolded, apprehension about the teaching machine reflected the growing cultural unease towards an increasingly technological, rather than humanistic, world order. Popular articles in the early 1960s, in addition to noting the revolutionary potential of programmed instruction, also repeatedly expressed the public's concern about the dehumanization of education through machine technology. Teachers and parents were especially sensitive to this issue. Boehm, writing for *Fortune* magazine in 1960, reported, 'the new method "dehumanizes" education by breaking the personal bond between teacher and student' (Boehm, 1960, p. 177). The associate editor of *Parents' Magazine* noted, '[I]t's hard to believe satisfactory substitutes will ever be found for a human teacher's warmth and encouragement, worldly experience, and ability to demonstrate subtle distinctions in taste' (Kreig, 1961, p. 78).

The social anomie of the late 1950s, with the subsequent rise of the counterculture and the humanistic movement, clearly signaled an increasing social apprehension about dehumanization, alienation, conformity, and loss of agency (Herman, 1992). In essence, the public's specific concerns about the teaching machine reveal an important feature of the historical moment in which the machines were introduced. An invention which could be seen as a mechanical antidote to human inefficiency, along with Skinner's emphasis on using the machines not to 'teach' in the traditional sense, but to bring the student's behavior under the control of the environment, may have met resistance in any period. However, as the 1960s unfolded, the temper of the times became increasingly inhospitable towards a technology that epitomized the automated mass society to which members of the counterculture movement were so vehemently opposed.

Popular articles about programmed instruction touched on themes of control, alienation, and conformity, even though the objective benefits of the technique were acknowledged and even praised. Some of these reactions highlighted the public's ambivalence towards achieving better educational results through the more rigid control of human behavior. For example, a reporter for *Popular Mechanics* remarked on his own sense of unease about the programs:

> One question in particular kept nagging at me as I talked with the people who are propagating machine teaching. The problem was articulated by teaching-machine expert Hugh Anderson, who told me, 'My wife was going through a programming sequence the other day in which the word "response" was sought repeatedly as the correct terminology ... She wanted to say "answer" instead. She resisted for a while, but soon she was automatically supplying the correct word so she could move on to the next point. Thus the programming had already shaped her behavior pattern.' (Bell, 1961, p. 157)

Skinner made no secret of the fact that programmed material was designed to shape verbal behavior, rather than 'teach' in any traditional sense of the word. In his 1958 article for *Science*, for example, he wrote, 'Teaching spelling is mainly a process of shaping complex forms of behavior' (Skinner, 1958, p. 971); and in his 1961 *Scientific American* article, 'Knowing how to read means exhibiting a behavioral repertory of great complexity' (Skinner, 1961b, p. 98).

The question of who would control the types of behaviors and responses that would be conditioned inevitably emerged. A writer for *Parents' Magazine* began her article: 'I'd been reading educational journals which questioned many aspects of automated instruction, not to mention newspaper warnings about robots taking over classrooms ... Was the dehumanized Brave New World really with us, I wondered. Is it 1984 already?' (Kreig, 1961, p. 45). Later, she quoted a 'leading authority' on audiovisual instruction who noted, 'Teaching machine programming is a social problem ... He who controls the programming heartland controls the educational system' (Kreig, 1961, p. 80). One reporter for *Time* referred to Skinner's method as 'Orwellian' ('Programed Learning,' 1961, p. 38).

Issues of freedom and control loomed large in the American psyche during the 1960s. Programmed instruction, more than any other educational technology, was premised on the control of student behavior. As Curti (1980) has noted, '[M]uch that was done in applying behavioral theory seemed to limit experience or to control it in questionable ways. This seemed evident in programmed instruction, teaching machines, and in time, the management ... of youths by behavior modification techniques' (p. 400).

Parents were also worried about the potential for social alienation if teaching machines filled the classroom. One parent at the Collegiate School for Boys in New York City, the site of one of the first experimental trials of the teaching machine, remarked, 'If they're just going to stick our boys behind machines, they might as well be in classes of fifty or even a hundred instead of a dozen' (as cited in Kreig, 1961, p. 76). William Ferry, president of the Center for the Study of Democratic Institutions, wrote that the teaching machine trend was responsible for the adoption of the 'totally wrong notion that an educational system is like a factory for producing steel plate or buttons ... The central claim is efficiency. Mass education, it is said, requires mass production. The result is already discernible, and may be called technication' ('The Critics Speak,' 1967, p. 56).

Conformity in thinking was also cited as a potential problem. Kreig (1961) noted, 'What will happen to the nurturing of creativity, imagination, and the intangibles of learning? Will reliance on programs discourage independent thinking and result in stultifying conformity among students and teachers alike?' (p. 80). Some felt that programmed instruction discouraged the development of the capacity to question, think critically, and consider multiple perspectives. A writer for *Fortune* magazine wrote:

> [T]he rigidity of structure that seems to be inherent in programed instruction may imply to students that there is indeed only one approach, one answer; yet what the students may need to learn most is that some questions may have more than one answer or no answer at all. (Silberman, 1966, p. 198)

Another writer summed this up as follows: 'A common criticism of programed instruction is that the answers required of students are too simple and too stereotyped, and that not enough individual freedom and diversity is permitted' (Suppes, 1967, p. 50). And on a more fatalistic note: 'If programing is used too extensively, moreover, it may prevent the development of intuitive and creative thinking or destroy such thinking when it appears' (Silberman, 1966, p. 198).

In many of these articles, yet another theme emerged: the need to harness technology in the service of a thoughtful educational philosophy. In January of 1967, *Saturday Review* published a series of articles in a section entitled 'Changing Directions in American Education.' In the article entitled 'What Tasks for the Schools?' the problem was framed this way:

> When we face the challenge of the new technology – how to employ for proper educational ends such instruments as television, teaching machines, or computer systems – our decisions must be made in the light of the total impact of instruction upon the individual, centering upon knowledge and the rational intellect but not violating the claims of the emotions and volition. (McMurrin, 1967, p. 40)

In addition to questioning whether the new technology could fulfil the claims of the emotions, apprehension about the creation of a technological order was likely increased by corporate America's annexation of the new technology. From 1962 to 1966, big business picked up on the profit potential of the largely untapped educational industry. A number of electronics companies bought or merged with publishing houses that made educational films, designed tests and programmed instructional materials, and produced other small educational instruments (see Ridgeway, 1966; Silberman, 1966).[15] The interest of big business in controlling this technology alarmed many. As a writer for *Christian Century* put it: '[We] must ask whether the thrust of business endangers the character and quality of education' ('Electronic Instruction: Blessing or Curse?' 1966, p. 1201). Simultaneously, large segments of the American population, especially its youth, expressed dissatisfaction with a society that was becoming increasingly corporatized and technocratic in its orientation.

As corporations seized control of the educational technology industry, and as society at large became increasingly dissatisfied with the techno-fervor of the 1950s, the appeal of programmed instruction and teaching machines dwindled. In the age of encounter groups, Esalen, and authenticity, automated education meted out by large corporations had to fight not only 'old-fashioned resistance to change' (Benjamin, 1988, p. 711) but also the tide of anti-technocratic sentiment that washed over society in the late 1960s. As one critic remarked, 'University students can see what is happening to them, and complain, and demonstrate. For this reason alone it would seem likely that technication will make its slowest inroads in the colleges and universities' (Ferry, as cited in 'The Critics Speak,' 1967, p. 57).

Again, Skinner could not have anticipated the complex interplay of factors that would influence the popular reception of his technology. He remained convinced of the value and potential of programmed instruction even after he stopped actively developing it himself. He was, however, skeptical of the use of computers as instructional devices. In an interview for *Forbes*, Skinner remarked disparagingly, 'Don't let the computer people sell you on their machines as teaching devices. It's a fad ... As a means of storing information, like a library ... or as part of school and classroom management systems, the computer can do a job. But as a teaching device it's ridiculous' ('Ice Cream for the Right Answers,' 1968, p. 46).

As Vargas and Vargas (1996) have noted, Skinner's concerns about education were, for him, more than a passing fad. He was perplexed by the laissez-faire approach of many of his educator colleagues who cavalierly accepted congratulations for a successful student's performance, but disavowed any responsibility for a poor student's failure to learn. He was encouraged by the hundreds of letters he received from parents, business people, and professional educators who, in looking for solutions to their problems, found a solution in programmed instruction. He repeatedly emphasized his intention that programmed instruction be used in addition to, rather than as a replacement for, human teachers.[16] His desire to create a better classroom was part and parcel of his desire to create a better world: 'Skinner's concerns [about education] fitted the utopian themes continually found in his writings. These themes inevitably addressed how a science of behavior could be applied to better the human condition' (Vargas and Vargas, 1996, p. 248).

Skinner's desire to better the human condition culminated in an impassioned plea for the application of behavioral principles to such problems as overpopulation, environmental degradation, energy depletion, and nuclear annihilation. As the inventor of the air crib and the teaching machine, Skinner had provoked considerable public debate. With the publication of *Beyond Freedom and Dignity*, however, the debate was about to become a national uproar.

Beyond Belief

The public furor over Skinner and his social message reached its highest point, and Skinner reached the height of his status as a public intellectual, following the publication of his best-selling *Beyond Freedom and Dignity* (*BFD*) in 1971. The main thesis of the book was that traditional notions of freedom and free will are illusions. Skinner argued that all behavior is con-trolled by subtle and complex systems of environmental contingencies. His prescription was that these contingencies must be recognized and deliber-ately manipulated through a technology of behavior if we are to improve our prospects for long-term physical, cultural, and social survival. He argued that this deliberate control would only be possible if we gave up our antiquated and sentimental belief in 'autonomous man' and embraced the science and technology of behavior.

Not surprisingly, Skinner's book struck a powerful chord in his popu-lar audiences. Most, though not all, responses were negative. In an inter-view for *Psychology Today* in 1972, Skinner reported that, by his estimates, about 80 per cent of reviews of *BFD* were negative (Hall, 1972).[17] In 1971 and 1972, five articles in the *New York Times* alone critiqued Skinner's attempt to draw out a social philosophy based on operant theory (see 'Is Freedom Obsolete,' 1971; Lehmann-Haupt, 1971; Reinhold, 1972; Sennett, 1971; Stevens, 1971). In one of these articles, Skinner's book was presented as 'an uninhibited assault on some of the Western world's most prized ideals' (Stevens, 1971, p. 29) which was sure to 'raise howls of opposition from the humanists and libertarians who have long opposed his behavioral psychology' (p. 29). In others, parallels were drawn between Skinner's vision in *BFD*, Orwell's *1984*, and Huxley's *Brave New World*. Concerns that the 'power over behavior' inherent in Skinner's technology might end up in the hands of a Stalin or a Hitler were reported.[18]

Readers of Skinner's book and the press coverage that ensued were quick to pick up on these powerful images. In an undated letter to Skinner, a young reader named Robert Newman expressed his con-cerns by sending Skinner the cover from his paperback copy of *BFD*, the back of which featured a photograph of Skinner which he had altered to produce a likeness of Hitler. In his letter he wrote, 'I think I would have burnt your book, but that had fascist overtones and besides, I wanted to show it to a few people first. You make me sick. How's that for subjectiv-ity?'[19] Another reader wrote, 'He sounds like a present day Hitler.'[20] And yet another likened Skinner's role to that of Nietzsche's in paving the way for fascism: 'Skinner's is the psychology of an amoral world ... One can only wonder if the bondage and indignities that ensued from Blond Europe's reading of Nietzsche will be matched when Redneck America gets around to reading Skinner.'[21]

References to fascism continued in a 1972 *New York Times* article entitled 'B.F. Skinner's Philosophy Fascist? Depends on How It's Used, He Says' (Reinhold, 1972). This article reported on a series of panel discussions on Skinner's work held at Yale University. The panel consisted of psychologists, politicians, and literary critics, among others. One panel member characterized Skinner's ideas as 'a kind of fascism without tears' (Reinhold, 1972, p. 41) and remarked that there was little room for the individuality of the artist and the poet in his vision. Skinner conceded that he, for one, would prefer the more peaceful and less troubled world made possible through behavioral engineering, even though he might have to give up the 'art of the past': 'I myself would choose to live in a world in which no one could understand what the devil was eating Dostoyevsky' (p. 41). Other readers offered their vehement objections to Skinner's work in their personal letters to him, or in letters to the editor of *Psychology Today*, which had printed excerpts from *BFD* in advance of the book's publication. Apparently, Skinner was surprised by the emotionality and vehemence of the negative reactions. In a letter to a colleague he wrote, 'The extraordinarily violent and negative reaction to my book has been a curious phenomena [*sic*] which I have not yet managed to put in perspective.'[22] Many of these letters contained impassioned, ad hominem attacks:

I have always considered you a fatuous, opinionated ass ... Quite obviously you are an apologist for totalitarianism. You seek an ant-heap culture, the abolition of all humanistic values, in a word, the destruction of the human spirit.[23]

Here's hoping that Dr. Skinner will be recognized soon as visibly insane and that his stay in a mental hospital ordered on the principle of behavior mod will enable him to feel right at home.[24]

I feel qualified to state that virtually every non-psychologist scholar on the university campus considers psychologists nuts. Your newest book substantiates this thought.[25]

Richard Sennett, a sociologist at New York University, reviewed the book for the *New York Times Book Review* (Sennett, 1971). In a somewhat different, although no less disparaging, take, he argued that Skinner, in adopting a new stance as social philosopher, was espousing a return to a less complicated way of life, a life in which hard work and asceticism were valued, and that he was using the technology of behavior to show

how this *personal* vision might be implemented. Sennett concluded, 'Hoping to revive the morality of a less complicated age ... he appears to understand so little, indeed to care so little, about society itself, that the reader comes totally to distrust him' (p. 18).

Skinner was upset by Sennett's criticism. In response, he wrote a letter to the editor of the *New York Times Book Review* in which he protested Sennett's misrepresentation of his position:

> Professor Sennett repeatedly accuses me of subscribing to examples I merely offer for discussion. I do not rail against sex; I discuss its role. I do not 'believe in hard work'; I argue that a culture must produce the goods it needs – but as pleasantly as possible ... I do not treat people as if they were living 'in a vacuum'; the defenders of autonomous man do that in their neglect of the environment. I do not overlook the 'social causes' of behavior; I devote three chapters to them ... How are we to explain Professor Sennett's extraordinary misreading?[26]

In other articles, Skinner's social vision was deemed such a threat to the American system of government that a review of Skinner's funding from the National Institute of Mental Health was suggested ('Freedom and Funding,' 1971). Congressman Cornelius Gallagher, in an article in the *New Republic*, was quoted as saying that Skinner 'is advancing ideas which threaten the future of our system of government by denigrating the American traditions of individualism, human dignity, and self-reliance' ('Misplaced Zeal,' 1972, p. 14). Despite the threats, however, Skinner did retain his funding. Spiro Agnew, at a Farm Bureau address in Chicago, remarked that this new 'behavioral thinking' is 'very dangerous, and it is completely at odds with our basic belief in the dignity and worth of the individual' ('Agnew's Blast at Behaviorism,' 1972, p. 4). Anthony Burgess, author of *A Clockwork Orange*, in an article for the *Listener*, wrote:

> B.F. Skinner, with his ability to believe that there is something *beyond* freedom and dignity, wants to see the death of autonomous man. He may or may not be right, but in terms of the Judaeo-Christian ethic that *A Clockwork Orange* tries to express, he is perpetrating a gross heresy. (Burgess, 1972, p. 198; italics in original)

Finally, Skinner's book and his obvious atheism also provoked a response from Christian readers. Many were worried about Skinner's soul and urged him, in true evangelical style, to get in touch with God:

Mr. Skinner, man will never find true happiness until he is reconciled to God his maker through Jesus Christ his Son. By mailing the enclosed card you will receive a free Bible Correspondence Course through which you can learn to have this happiness.[27]

Others were slightly more subtle, but nonetheless urged Skinner to embrace a higher being, and reassured him of his deliverance:

In denying God you are denying yourself and in denying yourself you are closing the door on fulfillment. If God to you means a church, a minister, a congregation, a set of outmoded rules and customs, yes, discard Him. But do not deny Him. Seek Him in a higher level – your level. He's there waiting for you.[28]

Clearly, Skinner's call for the death of 'autonomous man' and his proposal to use the science and technology of behavior to solve the world's most pressing problems succeeded in upsetting large segments of the American public on philosophical, political, ideological, and even religious grounds. *BFD* propelled Skinner from scientist and inventor to social philosopher. In doing so, it also exposed him to intense public scrutiny. This scrutiny was both professional and personal.

Skinner's Public Image

In reviewing these portrayals of Skinner and interpretations of his work, no simple characterization emerges. To some he was a modern father, an educational revolutionary, and a social prophet. To others, he was a negligent parent, an anti-humanist, even a fascist. As Skinner's biographer, historian Daniel Bjork, has written: 'To his most fervent opponents, Skinner was the Darth Vader of American psychology, perhaps even the Hitler of late-twentieth-century science itself ... For others, however, Skinner was the brilliant originator of radical behaviorism' (Bjork, 1993, p, xi). Although few if any of these wide-ranging characterizations were based on personal contact with Skinner, it is clear that attitudes towards him as a person were conflated with attitudes towards his theories, and vice versa. Skinner was not unaware of this phenomenon. Upon learning that well-known child psychologist Bruno Bettelheim was spreading the rumor that Skinner's second daughter, Deborah, had become psychotic as a result of being raised in the air crib, Skinner wrote him the following:

From time to time I have heard rumors that the daughter we raised in an
Air-Crib became psychotic. Recently I heard that you had mentioned this
... Quite apart from the accuracy of such a report, I must say I am always
surprised to hear it cited as if it had some bearing upon my theories. I
should suppose that no system of psychiatry would be evaluated in terms of
what has happened to the children of those who subscribe to it.[29]

In his failure to anticipate that public exposure would also bring public
scrutiny of his personal life and some degree of character assessment,
Skinner may have been naïve. Given that he was proposing a radical
reconceptualization of human nature and the redesign of cultural, social,
and political life, it was not surprising that the public became interested
in Skinner 'the man.' A writer from *Playboy*, to take one example, devoted
considerable verbiage to his assessment of Skinner's personality:

I find Skinner to be talkative but distant, and shy ... He does have a sense
of humor, but it is genteel and restrained. Me, I like people who laugh
from the ground up. Somehow I can't imagine him enjoying the sense of
touch or smell. Yet he is a nice, pleasant old guy, charming and cordial.
And then too, he has another kind of passion, the deep smoldering devo-
tion to the laboratory, the love of fact, statistic, insight and thesis. And I
have to remember that he labored for decades with no public recognition.
Now he is overwhelmed by violent personal attacks. (Pearce, 1972, p. 86).

On the one hand, Skinner may have been naïve in his belief that the
audiences for his work – even other psychologists – would be able to separate attitudes towards his science and philosophy from evaluations of his
personality. Moreover, he may have underestimated the degree to which
his public image would affect how people felt about his theories.
Although the relationship was a reciprocal one, one can't help but wonder whether Skinner's work, especially his later writing, might have been
better received if he had projected a warmer, more emotional persona.[30]
He was not unaware of his public image. In a letter to a friend who had
given him feedback on his 'Sketch for an Autobiography,' he wrote back:

I shall keep your comments on the Autobiography in my file for careful
review ... I have already been told that I need to get some emotion into it
to counteract my very bad public image. It pleases me to find that you
thought some parts of the Sketch were 'very warm.' I can also easily hear
you chuckling at the humerous [sic] parts.[31]

On the other hand, perhaps it is unfair to expect Skinner to play up to his audiences in this way. After all, he was not, in his own mind, primarily a celebrity. He was primarily a psychologist who believed strongly in his science, the philosophy behind it, and its applicability to everyday life – including his own. He held unwaveringly to the conviction that his life, his behavior, the 'self' that was Skinner, was a product of his phylogenic and ontogenic learning history, and nothing more. It would have been extremely duplicitous for Skinner to have behaved or professed otherwise; to do so would have, at least from his perspective, undermined his theories. As he remarked in an interview after completing the third volume of his autobiography, "If I am right about human behavior I have written the autobiography of a nonperson" (Skinner, 1983b, p. 32). In another reverse solipsism, a writer for *Time* magazine noted, 'He is one of the most formidable minds ever devoted to the notion that mind itself is unimportant' (Lee, 1983, p. 43).

Certainly the perception that Skinner 'lived behaviorism' had an impact on the conflation of attitudes towards him personally and his work generally. As a writer for *Science Digest* observed: 'Once in a while, a scientist becomes so committed to his theories that they color every aspect of his life. B.F. Skinner, the prominent Harvard psychologist, now 78, lives behaviorism ...' ('Utopia or Disaster,' 1983, p. 14). I would argue, however, that this conflation was more problematic for Skinner than for other visible scientists because of the nature of his science. He was proposing a science of human behavior, not a science of subatomic particles, chemical reactions, or Petri dishes. The same qualities that the public admired in their physicists, chemists, and biologists were qualities used pejoratively to describe Skinner. He was described by his critics as 'the archetype of the cold-blooded scientist for whom man is simply a machine' (Rice, 1968, p. 27). And while the public generally lauded physical scientists for having 'minds set apart and bodies detached from their hearts' (La Follette, 1990, p. 69), Skinner was singled out for his apparent lack of feeling and humanity. A writer for *McCall's* put it this way: 'On the evidence of his legendary career, Skinner is an enemy of sentiment ... This quality, so endearing in most people, is somehow incongruous in a sixty-seven-year-old scientist who believes he has found a way to control the behavior of the human race ...' (McCarry, 1971, p. 35).

As a psychologist, Skinner was expected (unlike other scientists) to have mind and heart firmly connected. By contrast (and to show you can't win either way), Fuller (1982), in an article examining the reception of Carl Rogers and his client-centered approach in American culture, has written:

No doubt [Rogers's] reluctance to reduce human personality to a strictly deterministic model has seriously equivocated the degree to which his theories have been perceived as properly belonging to scientific psychology. It is thus all the more tempting to interpret the overall popularity of his psychological writings as owing to their resonance with cultural forces that are themselves independent of the institutional mechanisms of psychological science. (P. 31).

So although Skinner's work embraced scientism, it occasionally ran amok of the cultural forces to which Fuller refers. It was this overwhelming scientism – as applied to the human science of psychology – that provoked much of the public criticism of Skinner's views. One reader of *BFD* expressed it this way: 'His assumption that psychology is comparable to exact physical science is fallacious. He may *hope* it to be, and say that it *ought* to be, but facts have yet to verify this [italics in original].'[32]

Interestingly, the reception of Freud's theories mirrors the dilemma that Fuller outlined for Rogers. Although criticized as lacking any scientific basis, Freud's theories have nonetheless resonated strongly with people's experiences of their own lives. As a journalist from the *Washington Post* put it, '[P]sychoanalysis has won its following – both among the population at large and among artists and intellectuals – precisely because, unlike academic psychology, it speaks to the felt problems of human life and says things that are far from self-evident' (Robinson, 1983, p. 7).

Skinner himself, in literally embodying his science, ran into serious trouble with his public image. In venturing beyond the safe confines of his Harvard laboratory, he found himself up against an entrenched refusal to re-envision the human subject as scientific object. Despite this cultural opposition, there remained a large and receptive opening for Skinner's behavioral engineering. This opening, as I and others have already suggested, was the powerful American penchant for making and remaking the environment. As anthropologist-historian Rebecca Lemov has remarked, the social science of which Skinner's behaviorism formed a part was 'one that could only have emerged out of the peculiar life-sized Petri dish where American ambition, open space, and can-do approach combined in the agar of scientific advance' (Lemov, 2005, p. 5). It would fall to Skinner's students and colleagues, working steadily in the shadow of his expanding public persona, to take advantage of this opening and fully exploit the potential of a technology of behavior. First, however, Skinner's science of behavior, established with rats and pigeons, would have to become the science of *human* behavior.

chapter 2

From Pigeons to People:
Constructing the Human Skinner Box

I certainly do not recommend working with the 'fewest possible' animals. On the other hand there are important strategic decisions to be made. Human behavior is the subject of greatest interest and if I had had the facilities I should have used species closer to it than rat or pigeon. But I should not have felt it necessary to cover the waterfront any more than an immunologist would feel it necessary to cover immunological processes in a very large number of species.[1]

For critics, the fact that Skinner's own basic experimental work was conducted almost exclusively with rats and pigeons in the rigidly controlled environment of the operant chamber became problematic when he and his followers extended his principles to the problems of human beings in the real world. Some were skeptical on purely scientific grounds, arguing that without the appropriate studies Skinner could not assume that his findings would replicate with humans under very different conditions. Others had a more emotional reaction. These critics objected to the implied equivalence of lower organisms and human beings that they discerned in Skinner's work. For example, one aspiring poet parodied Skinner in verse:

Dr. Skinner took a rat,
And in his easy chair he sat,
And held the rodent on his knees,
And gave each little paw a squeeze.
And said, 'Oh mirror of mankind,
Whose ways so accurately I find
Reflect the masses – Yet I say

Not *every* man behaves that way,
For some, in matters of religion,
Most nearly imitate the pigeon ...[2]

Despite the fact that Skinner himself never undertook an experimental analysis of *human* behavior, several of his colleagues and students did construct analogues of the operant chamber for use with human subjects. In essence, these researchers created human-sized Skinner boxes complete with manipulanda, delivery chutes, reinforcers, and cumulative recorders. These were men (largely) who were familiar with Skinner's basic methods and envisioned how to apply them to the scientific study of human behavior. If Skinner's system had in fact proceeded linearly from basic research with animals, to basic research with humans, to human application, these men would be responsible for bridging Skinner's experimental principles with animals to applied work with humans. As we shall see, however, this process did not proceed linearly, and the relations between the experimentalists and the 'behavior shapers,' as they became known in the popular press (see Goodall, 1972), were in many cases somewhat distant.

In this chapter, I survey three examples of work undertaken inside human-sized Skinner boxes. In each example, the ultimate goals for the researcher were observation, measurement, and recording of human behavior, not behavior change. However, through such projects, the Skinner box expanded both physically and conceptually. Although these researchers remained 'within the box' so to speak, they did take a few tentative steps beyond the box, and either intentionally or unintentionally moved Skinner's system closer to the realm of full-blown application. In discussing their work, I also move this account beyond the box by moving beyond Skinner himself to focus on those who worked with him and were influenced by him. First, I discuss Charles Ferster's work with autistic children at the Indiana University Medical Center. Then I move to Ogden Lindsley's research with chronic schizophrenics at Metropolitan State Hospital. Finally, and moving ever-closer to applied work, I survey Sidney Bijou's studies of child behavior in his Mobile Child Study Laboratory. Each of these men extended the use of the free operant method[3] to human beings by constructing rooms that closely resembled the operant chambers used in experiments with pigeons and rats.

Although there are many other examples of work in human-sized Skinner boxes,[4] these three case studies demonstrate that Skinner's neglect of the area did not deter other researchers from employing humans as their subject of greatest interest. In one particularly bizarre study (Ader and Tatum, 1961), human subjects were led, with no instructions, into a cubicle where they had to press a lever to delay the onset of electric shock. Instead of lever-pressing, half of the subjects chose instead to disconnect the electrodes and walk out of the experiment – arguably a more effective avoidance procedure! Although this body of research established a tradition of basic studies of human operant behavior, this tradition was soon overshadowed by the dominance of applied behavior analysis throughout the 1960s and 1970s. However, the area experienced a renaissance in the 1980s (Baron and Perone, 1982; Buskist and Miller, 1982; Miller, 1983). The experimental analysis of human behavior, or EAHB, has now been institutionalized as a Special Interest Group of the burgeoning Association for Behavior Analysis International.

But well before this, in their efforts to 'cover the waterfront,' Skinnerian researchers selected many species for experimentation in operant chambers or similar kinds of apparatus, including dogs, primates, and even goldfish.[5] Prior to working with humans, Skinner's colleague Charles Ferster spent two years working with chimpanzees at the Yerkes Laboratories of Primate Biology in Orange Park, Florida. Although Ferster's time at Orange Park was controversial, his studies there did extend findings on schedules of reinforcement in pigeons to a species closer to our own. As Skinner remarked in a letter written soon after Ferster arrived at Orange Park, 'All the stuff about the chimps sounds fascinating and I look forward to further reports.'[6] An examination of Ferster's work over the first decade of his career reveals a progression from pigeon to chimpanzee to human using the free operant method and the physically expanding Skinner box to extend the operant project. Skinner and Ferster met at Skinner's influential Pigeon Lab and were good friends until Ferster's untimely death in 1981 at the age of fifty-nine.

Charles Ferster and the Harvard Pigeon Lab

Charles Ferster was a twenty-seven-year-old graduate student at Columbia University in the fall of 1949 when he first heard about an opportunity to work with Skinner. Columbia was a natural place for Skinner to come looking for help: the university was a hotbed of operant psychology. Fred Keller, Skinner's colleague and close friend since their graduate school days together at Harvard, was on faculty there and had just completed his seminal text *Principles of Psychology* with Nat Schoenfeld. Under their influence, a bevy of students had become fascinated with the operant approach. As Ferster later recalled of the atmosphere at Columbia, 'Everyone had conditioned a rat, read *Walden Two*, and most were impatient to try out a science of behavior. Some students fantasied a new Institute for Operant Behavior ... Others dreamed of an actual planned community modeled after *Walden Two* ...' (Ferster, 2002/1970, p. 303).

So when Ferster heard that Skinner was looking for a researcher to join his team, he immediately made an appointment for an interview and hopped on the midnight train from New York to Boston. Arriving at six in the morning, he 'wandered around Harvard Square nervously' until what he thought would be a 'respectable hour to appear at Skinner's office' (Ferster, 2002/1970, p. 303). After a casual meeting consisting of sodas and a tour of the labyrinthine basement of Memorial Hall, Ferster was hired and asked to return February 1st to become an official staff member of the Pigeon Lab.[7] He rushed back to Columbia, executed some rather hurried dissertation research to meet his deadline, and arrived at Harvard in the winter of 1950 to take up his post.

Ferster's initial weeks at the laboratory were consumed with adjusting equipment, tweaking experimental procedures, examining data, and organizing the incredible array of tools, parts, devices, and gadgets that served the needs of the lab members. Because the lab was set up to record the cumulative rates of pigeon-pecking in dozens of operant chambers, most of the daily discussions in 'Grand Rounds' centered around apparatus design and construction. All experimental sessions were completely automated and could last up to ten hours. Over time, each cumulative recorder had to stand up to literally billions of pigeon pecks. Thousands of feet of cumulative curves were generated. As Ferster emphasized in a manner reminiscent of Skinner's 1956 *Case Study in Scientific Method*, 'The physical arrangements of the laboratory, the supplies, the equipment and the shop were important factors in determining the kind of research that went on' (Ferster, 2002/ 1970, p. 305). Indeed, this experience constructing and servicing cumulative recorders, programmers, and food magazines in a well-stocked and physically reinforcing laboratory environment influenced Ferster more than he realized at the time. He later remarked that it taught him how to run a laboratory, how to design experiments, and how to actually *conceptualize* research problems. Not surprisingly, Ferster would use the Pigeon Lab experiments as models for his future work with primates and human subjects.

Orange Park: The Primate Experience

After what he described as an intense and rewarding five-year collaboration with Skinner which resulted in their co-authored book *Schedules of*

Reinforcement,[8] Ferster accepted an invitation facilitated by Karl Pribram to work at the Yerkes Laboratories of Primate Biology in Orange Park, Florida. Here was a chance to apply what he had learned in the Pigeon Lab to the study of primate behavior. He arrived in July of 1955 immediately after Henry Nissen had assumed the directorship of the facility. Ferster quickly added two staff members to his team – Roger Kelleher and John Falk – and the trio conducted a series of studies on schedules of reinforcement, conditioned reinforcement, and discrimination learning in chimpanzees. The experimental procedures they devised for working with the chimps drew heavily on Ferster's experience in the Pigeon Lab, and orders for equipment to construct experimental spaces for the primates were frequent. In one published report, Ferster remarked of the methodological similarities – 'The specific experimental conditions were similar to those already described for the pigeon' (Ferster, 1957, p. 1090) – although they were presumably executed on a somewhat larger scale. Instead of pecking a key to get grain, the chimps would press a key to get a portion of chow. At one point, Ferster became nostalgic 'for the old days when the s [subject] could be lifted out of the operant chamber.'[9]

The importation of *some* of the Pigeon Lab methods, however, met with resistance. Of considerable controversy was the practice of using food deprivation to increase the chimps' motivation to work on the reinforcement schedules. At Orange Park, Ferster and his operant colleagues typically reduced the chimps to 80 per cent of free-feeding weight in order to get them to work. This had been standard practice in the Pigeon Lab. Most non-operant researchers, however, felt this was both unnecessary and inhumane (see Dewsbury, 2003, for an account of these disagreements). For his part, Ferster felt that some of the practices used by other scientists at the Yerkes Labs were themselves misguided. In a letter to Skinner written a few months after his arrival, Ferster noted:

> As usual the techniques of handling the animals involve aversive control exclusively. A stream of water from a hose, a toy soaked in kerosene at the end of a stick are frequently used to get them into a small carrying crate for weighing on the big scale, for example. My animals compete to get into the box. How something as simple as putting food in the box can elude them, I can't conceive ... I think it's the pure enjoyment of punishing the animals that makes them use aversive control.[10]

Despite the friction between the operant and non-operant scientists, it was an intensely productive period for Ferster's group, resulting in about a dozen published articles over the course of his short tenure there (e.g., Falk, 1958; Ferster, 1958; Kelleher, 1957). In the end, deteriorating collegial relationships prompted a move, and Ferster left Orange Park in the summer of 1957, effectively ending the brief period of operant psychology at the 'Monkey Farm.'[11]

From Chimps to Children

From 1957 until 1962, Ferster worked at the Indiana University Medical Center, where he took a position at the Institute of Psychiatric Research as a professor and 'Principal Investigator of Experimental Psychology.'[12] At Indiana he finally had the opportunity to work with human beings. His subjects were autistic children hospitalized at the Institute. After his tenure at the pigeon and primate labs, how did Ferster conceptualize his research problems when working with humans?

In what had now become standard operating procedure, Ferster decided to investigate operant behavior in autistic children by importing the techniques of food deprivation, key pressing, automated reinforcer delivery, and continuous measurement that he had used in his previous work. But, given that these were children and not chimps, how was food deprivation operationalized? Still convinced that deprivation was necessary to motivate responding, he explained in one research report that it was accomplished by denying children snacks between meals (Ferster and DeMyer, 1962, p. 93).

The experimental space designed for research with these children was a room containing a variety of devices necessary for the free operant method: a response console where the child subject could press a key and receive a coin, a number of vending machines where the child could deposit coins and receive a variety of reinforcers, and a matching-to-sample apparatus.[13] Along one wall was a one-way mirror for observation. In a typical experiment, each child was oriented to the room by an attendant, and then was left alone 'during the entire experimental procedure' (Ferster and DeMyer, 1962, p. 93), which lasted from one to three hours, depending on the subject. There were no exceptions to this practice except during the most extreme tantrums. One unintended outcome was that when a child 'was locked in an experimental space daily for over a year,' the 'frequency of tantrums and atavisms declined continuously ... until they almost disappeared' (Ferster, 1961, p. 440). Ferster took this as convincing proof of the operant nature of several autistic behaviors, with social attention serving as the reinforcer in the child's natural environment.

In terms of key-pressing, Ferster explicitly compared the children's performance to the performance of other species: 'When coins were delivered by pressing a simple key the pattern of emission of the child's behavior was like that normally occurring under similar reinforcement conditions in other species' (Ferster and DeMyer, 1962, p. 94). As in the pigeon and primate labs, graphic records of cumulative curves were generated and examined. The results, according to one report, showed that it was possible to 'bring the behavior of these children under the close control of an artificial environment' (ibid., p. 97), indicating that despite their other deficits, autistic children were not much different from pigeons and chimps in their ability to generate lawful response rates. Also not unlike his previous subjects, the children were tested extensively, sometimes spending over two hundred sessions in the room-sized Skinner box.

Ferster concluded his reports of these experimental analyses with firm statements about the basic rather than applied nature of the work: 'We do not consider these techniques as attempts at rehabilitation but rather as experimental analyses of the actual and potential repertoires of these children' (Ferster and DeMyer, 1962, p. 97); and 'This experimental program is not viewed as an attempt at carrying out psychotherapy' (Ferster and DeMyer, 1961, p. 344). Nonetheless, he did indicate that results might prove useful in efforts to develop increased social behaviors in the children, or as baseline measurements to evaluate drug effects. This latter technique, in fact, was being used by another Pigeon Lab alumnus, Ogden Lindsley.

Ogden Lindsley: Dogs, Drugs, and Rates of Response

Ogden Lindsley was a frequent participant in the Pigeon Staff meetings from 1951 to 1964, first as a graduate student and then as a postdoctoral researcher. As he later put it, 'Much, much more than pigeon research happened in the west end of Harvard's Memorial Hall basement in the early 1950s' (Lindsley, 2002, p. 385).[14] Lindsley entered psychology after a harrowing experience as a German prisoner of war, whereupon he had vowed to spend the rest of his life having fun and studying people. But for Lindsley, as for Ferster, research with people did not happen right away. For his dissertation with Skinner, Lindsley designed and built the first Skinner box for dogs.

To get him started on his dissertation research, Skinner directed Lindsley to Walter Jetter at the Boston University Medical School, who held a grant from the Atomic Energy Commission to study the effects of irradiation on the physiology, exercise, and behavior of beagles. To study the effects of irradiation on behavior, Lindsley designed an operant chamber in which the dogs were required to paw-press a panel for portions of raw hamburger. Using sixty-three two-year-old male beagles, Lindsley established reliable variable-interval response rates and then taught the dogs to stop pressing the panel when a light flashed and when a buzzer signaled an aversively loud horn blast. He then examined the effects of various drugs on the operant response rates, visual discrimination, and conditioned suppression that he had established.

After the effects of varying doses of alcohol, Nembutal, and methamphetamine were established for calibration purposes, the dogs were subjected to total body irradiation at a level that killed half of them over a period of fifteen days as their white cell counts decreased. Lindsley later remarked of the dogs's demise, 'Invading organisms go through a mammal so fast when there's no white cells you can't believe it' (Lindsley, 2004, interview with the author). The other half of the dogs recovered gradually. Both groups were extensively tested immediately after irradiation and over the fifteen-day period, not only for the effects of the irradiation on their operant behavior, but also on their maze-running performance. Lindsley found that physically ill dogs demonstrated lower response rates, but well-preserved visual discrimination and conditioned suppression. Although the practical implications of these findings were not clear, Lindsley felt that the beagle experiments were personally worthwhile: 'From our free operant research I was strongly rewarded for apparatus design and procedure innovation. I had introduced a new species to the free operant! … This strengthened my resolve to use the free operant with people' (Lindsley, 2001, pp. 137–8).

Despite his enthusiasm for the beagle work, Lindsley was still more interested in human than dog behavior. His opportunity to study humans came again as a result of Skinner's connections. During the course of their meetings to discuss Lindsley's dissertation research, they often strayed from the topic of beagle behavior to the topic of schizophrenia. Lindsley became fascinated by the possible operant nature of psychotic behavior. As he reported in a retrospective account:

Fascinated, I promised Fred [Skinner] that if he could get funds, I would give human free operant research with psychotics five years of my life. If it didn't pan out, my parachute plan was to go to Ringling Brothers Circus and shape Gargantua the gorilla to play a piano and simple card games. I ended up spending eleven and a half years studying psychotics from the back wards of Metropolitan State Hospital. (Lindsley, 2001, p. 138).

In 1952, Skinner met Harry Solomon, head of the Department of Psychiatry at Harvard and director of the Boston Psychopathic Hospital. Solomon was known to be theoretically open-minded even though psychoanalytic thinking was then hegemonic in psychiatry. He was immediately interested in Skinner's proposal to establish a human operant lab to study psychotic behavior. He persuaded William McLaughlin, the superintendent of Metropolitan State Hospital in Waltham, Massachusetts, to give Skinner and his colleagues space for a laboratory.[15] With a physical location secured, Skinner patched together funds from the Office of Naval Research, the Rockefeller Foundation, and the Milton Fund of Harvard University, and put Lindsley in charge of the project.

In June of 1953, Lindsley's dream of studying people was realized. The 'Experimental Analysis of the Behavior of Psychotic Patients' set up shop in an abandoned hydrotherapy unit in the basement of the hospital. Lindsley quickly converted the unit into a state-of-the-art experimental space, including two six-foot-square operant chambers equipped with plunger operanda and magazine delivery chutes designed to administer a variety of reinforcements to human subjects.[16] The plungers were connected through programming relays and timers to cumulative recorders situated in a hallway adjacent to the experimental rooms, which Lindsley came to call 'Apparatus Alley.' Eventually, the lab became known as the Harvard Medical School Behavior Research Laboratory.

The early research undertaken at the Behavior Research Laboratory clearly drew upon the free operant method used with other organisms and practiced par excellence in the Pigeon Lab. In one of their first publications, Lindsley and Skinner described their method of introducing their subjects – male psychiatric patients hospitalized an average of seventeen years – to the experimental situation. Patients were brought down to the laboratory and were shown a variety of potential reinforcers, including candy, cigarettes, and coins. They were prompted to select their preferred reinforcer. For some patients, none of these seemed to have any reinforcing value, and so more options were introduced, including projecting 'short exposures of interesting pictures' – actually photos of pin-up girls – onto a wall (Skinner, Solomon, and Lindsley, 1954, p. 403).

Subjects were then led to the experimental room, where, in the case of severely catatonic patients, they were shown how to operate the plunger that would deliver the reinforcer, or, in the case of better-functioning patients, were allowed to explore the room freely until plunger-pulling was emitted. With effective reinforcers established and the operant response introduced, two schedules of reinforcement were investigated – a one-minute variable interval schedule in which plunger-pulling was reinforced on average once every minute, and a fixed-ratio of twenty, in which every twentieth response was reinforced. Skinner and Lindsley concluded that the effects of different schedules of reinforcement on the behavior of their schizophrenic subjects were orderly and similar to those found in rats, pigeons, and dogs. They recommended further study, specifically using these response rates as baselines for investigating the moment-to-moment effects of drugs (Skinner, Solomon, and Lindsley, 1954).

Drugs and Behavior in the Box

Skinner's direct involvement with the Behavior Research Laboratory (BRL) waned by the late 1950s, but by this time Ogden Lindsley had earned his PhD and assumed full directorship of the lab. Funds continued to pour in from the National Institute of Mental Health (NIMH), both to support the general operations of the BRL and for specific projects. It was not a cheap operation. In a letter to the chief of the Research Grants and Fellowships Branch of the NIMH, Philip Sapir, Skinner wrote that the first two rooms had cost about $10,000 each to build and equip. With funds from the NIMH, he and Lindsley hoped to construct five additional experimental rooms, at the cost of about $7,000 each. Skinner justified the expenditures by highlighting the volume of data that could be collected and the relative efficiency (and superiority) of automatically recorded data over personal observation:

> The anticipated total number of recorded hours of behavior is of the order of 10,000 per year, thanks to the automatic nature of the equipment. This amounts to about $5.00 per hour, which seems a reasonable figure compared with the cost of recording, organizing, and publishing comparable data obtained through personal observation. Our figures for equipment and supplies of $26,000 and $18,000 respectively for two years might be judged in comparison with the salaries of competent observers who would be needed to make what would probably be an inferior record of the same behavior.[17]

Evidently, Skinner was persuasive. The NIMH granted two years of support for the BRL: $30,000 for the first year and $20,000 for the second.[18] As Skinner remarked to Harry Solomon upon receiving the news, 'Now we are in business.'[19]

From 1958 to 1965, Lindsley received additional NIMH grants for projects entitled 'Screening Potential Stimulants on Inactive Psychotics' and 'Drug-Sensitive Free-Operant Measures of Psychosis.' The late 1950s and early 1960s were truly a golden age for operant research on drug effects (see Laties, 2003). In the last volume of his autobiography, Skinner remarked of this period:

> Thanks mainly to Joe Brady, who was actively promoting the experimental analysis of behavior in the assessment and study of drugs, almost all the large ethical pharmaceutical companies had set up operant laboratories. Advertisements for new drugs began to show cumulative recorders, and *Life* magazine ran a full-page picture in color of an unboxed rat pressing a lever surrounded by racks of relays and timers. (Skinner, 1983a, p. 116)

Although the rats in *Life* were unboxed, the same could not be said of Lindsley's human subjects. In fact, his human-sized Skinner boxes were becoming increasingly elaborate. Lindsley equipped each room with electrical mats to record pacing and mounted voice-operated relays on the ceiling to record vocal hallucinations. In a 1962 article, Lindsley outlined results from four case studies investigating both the immediate and chronic effects of three drug compounds on plunger-pulling behavior reinforced on a one-minute variable interval schedule. Extensive pre-experimental baseline records were established for each subject in the room-sized Skinner boxes. The effects of the drug compounds were then evaluated according to whether they affected the rate of vocal hallucinatory behavior and plunger-pulling. With typical enthusiasm Lindsley noted, 'The technique of direct, continuous, and simultaneous recording of symptomatic and nonsymptomatic responding is the most sensitive index we have yet developed for screening psychotherapeutic compounds' (Lindsley, 1962, p. 378). The genius lay in the method, and the method was intimately tied to the apparatus.

Sometimes, however, the apparatus could not withstand the subjects' behavior. To overcome the effects of occasional outbursts of violence during the experimental sessions, Lindsley and his colleagues designed indestructible equipment. Describing the interior of an experimental room at the end of a one-hour session during which a violent patient had a 'destructive episode,' Lindsley noted proudly, 'The patient broke his chair against the work panel, but did not harm our indestructible panel' (Lindsley, 2001, p. 141).

Longevity, as well as indestructibility, was no doubt an issue. Lindsley's 'core group' of fifty male chronic psychotic patients took part in daily sessions for as long as ten years. However, in 1965, due to changes in funding practices and the increasing expense of running the lab, the BRL closed its doors.[20] During the course of its eleven-year tenure, hundreds of students, post-doctoral researchers, and colleagues had visited the lab or conducted research there. Among these visitors and researchers were many who went on to make pioneering contributions in behavioral pharmacology, education, and treatment. Teodoro Ayllon and Nathan Azrin, who later collaborated on the first token economy program for hospitalized psychiatric patients, both spent time at the lab. Lindsley reported that Sidney Bijou visited the BRL in April 1957, November 1961, and April 1962, and went on to build a similar laboratory for children at the University of Washington (Lindsley, 2001, p. 149). Although the BRL was devoted to basic research, it served a pivotal role in the expansion of behavior analysis beyond its experimental origins.

Sidney Bijou: A Clinical Experimentalist

Ferster and Lindsley conducted their human operant research with autistic and schizophrenic patients committed to in-patient psychiatric wards. Although neither man had ever worked with psychiatric patients or had any clinical experience, each was primarily interested in extending the free operant method to other species and generating experimental results. They had access to these relatively captive populations partly through their connections, and partly because these were individuals who were deemed beyond help and were powerless to make their own decisions about whether or not to participate. In an era before well-established ethical review procedures and institutional review boards, these patient populations were, so to speak, up for grabs. For their part, Ferster and Lindsley imported or adapted their techniques to suit the situation, but did not view the idiosyncrasies of their particular subjects as detracting from their research aims. Nor did they intend their studies as attempts at therapy. Perhaps surprisingly, despite Sidney Bijou's clinical background, he extended the free operant situation to studies of normal children, leaving extensions to 'clinical' populations to his students and colleagues.

Bijou began his training in the 1930s as a clinical psychologist, receiving his master's degree at Columbia in 1937 with Henry Garrett, and his doctorate at the University of Iowa in 1941 (Bijou, 2001; Krasner, 1977). Between his degrees he took a position at the Delaware State Mental Hygiene Clinic near Wilmington. In what was typical of psychologists' roles at the time, this job mainly involved psychological testing, report-writing, and diagnostic consultation. However, while at Delaware he also worked closely with Joseph Jastak to develop the Wide Range Achievement Test of academic skills, which remains a widely used test to this day. Bijou then applied to do a PhD at Iowa on the recommendation that he work with Kurt Lewin, who was described to him by G.W. Hartmann at Teachers College as 'a gifted person who was going to do great things in the field of child development' (Bijou, in Wesolowski, 2002, p. 17).

Bijou's affiliation with Lewin, however, did not pan out. Unbeknownst to Bijou, Lewin was on the staff of the Iowa Child Welfare Research Station and was not a member of the department of psychology where Bijou was registered (see Krasner, 1977). So, after a rather circuitous route, Bijou actually ended up working with noted learning theorist Kenneth Spence, who became not only his advisor but also a close friend. As Bijou remarked of his doctoral training: 'Among the highlights of my training at Iowa were Spence's two-semester course in animal learning and conditioning and his informal seminar, The Monday Night Group' (Bijou, 2001, p. 107). In the Monday Night Group, major topics included a chapter-by-chapter review of Clark Hull's manuscript for *Principles of Behavior*, Gustav Bergmann's course on logical positivism, and statistics, research design, and systematic psychology.

After completing his doctorate with a dissertation on experimental neurosis in rats, Bijou spent two years at a residential school for developmentally retarded children, and three years in military service. When he was ready to apply for academic positions in 1946, Skinner was chair of the Indiana University Psychology Department and the Pigeon Lab was not yet born. Bijou was about to start 'the second phase' of his experience and training (Bijou, 2001, p. 108).

As the chair at Indiana, Skinner needed a director for the newly established clinical program. He was looking for someone with an experimental-learning background and clinical experience. Bijou was perfect: his training with Spence provided him with the experimental-learning qualification, and his work at Delaware and in the military attested to his clinical experience. Bijou accepted Skinner's offer to join the department. It would be a short although lively appointment. At Indiana, Skinnerian, Hullian, and Kantorian views all jockeyed for position. Debates were heated and intellectually stimulating. As Bijou noted of his acquaintance with Skinner in this period, 'Skinner knew I was oriented toward Hullian learning theory through my training with Spence but did not "push" his view' (Bijou, in Wesolowski, 2002, p. 17).

Despite this congenial and exciting environment, neither Skinner nor Bijou lingered long at Indiana. Skinner left just two years after Bijou's arrival to take a permanent appointment at his alma mater, Harvard University, where he immediately set up the Pigeon Lab. In 1948, Bijou left Indiana, too, but headed west instead. He accepted a position at the University of Washington as associate professor and director of the Institute of Child Development (ICD). When he arrived, the institute consisted of a two-room clinic housed within the Psychology Department where children were administered psychological tests. Bijou had something different in mind. He envisioned a research organization consisting of a clinic, a preschool, and a child study unit. In 1950, he realized his vision and a new Institute was opened. It included a child development clinic, a two-unit nursery school, and a research laboratory. To appreciate the magnitude of both the physical and theoretical shifts that occurred under Bijou, consider the recollection of Eileen Allen, one of the psychologists at the precursor of what became the ICD nursery school:

> The ICD Nursery School, as we so fondly called it, was housed in a two-storey frame building built in 1905 for the Alaska-Yukon Exposition ... The philosophy was primarily developmental à la Gesell with strong undertones of Freud ... This was to change dramatically, however, when we became the Developmental Psychology Laboratory Preschool. Under the leadership of Bijou, Baer, and Wolf, the preschool teaching staff were converted from a psychodynamic, genetic, and biological determinism to full blown learning theory / behaviorism à la Skinner. Within a couple of years, we were publishing ground-breaking studies carried out in the naturalistic environment of the preschool classroom.[21]

Yet despite Bijou's exposure to Skinner at Indiana, and Allen's assessment of the preschool's Skinnerian conversion, when Bijou first arrived at the ICD he had not yet committed himself completely to Skinner. His reading of Hull had influenced him deeply, and in his new Institute he hoped to launch a series of studies testing Hullian learning principles with individual children. The challenges of designing the type of experiment he had in mind, however, soon defeated him, and he 'turned to the only other procedure I knew – Skinner's operant conditioning model' (Bijou, 2001, p. 110).

A Skinner Box on Wheels

Perhaps because of his diverse training, theoretical eclecticism, and child development background, Bijou did not automatically assume that his developmental colleagues would be convinced of the value of the free operant method with children. In his earliest publications, he tried to convince his readers that 'a systematic laboratory approach' had much to offer a field where studies 'in the natural setting' were often viewed as more meaningful (Bijou, 1955, p. 161). He advocated the use of the operant conditioning situation as a 'promising beginning point' for such a systematic approach, noting that relationships based on animal studies needed to be tested with human subjects before generalizations could be made and explaining that 'a methodology of this kind ... should enable one to study problems and behavior processes in children by relating the direct effect of one variable upon another' (Bijou, 1957, p. 243).

To create an operant conditioning situation for preschool children, Bijou, like Ferster and Lindsley, took inspiration from the animal laboratory: 'I wanted a method that would do what we had been doing in the animal laboratory ... I explored laboratory procedures that would be comparable in methodology to the animal research situation. I started with a ball-drop response ...' (Bijou, in Krasner, 1977, p. 590). Bijou began by constructing a simple piece of apparatus in which the child could get trinkets by placing a ball in a hole. This homemade device had a number of practical and technical limitations. For example, it was taking children too long to manipulate the ball and they would occasionally drop it, leading to response-rate anomalies. The operant response was too complex, although the device was interesting for the children because it was similar to toys they already knew. A different approach – and a different apparatus – was required.

In the next iteration of his operant conditioning situation, Bijou replaced ball-dropping with lever-pressing (the lever was constructed out of a handle grip for the squeezer of an O-Cedar sponge mop), and the box with the lever was painted with the face and head of a clown to make it child-friendly. A cumulative recorder was attached to the lever, and trinkets were delivered directly to the child via a delivery chute. In Bijou's revised set-up, a table with these devices was placed in a room with other toys and a one-way mirror. In a typical experiment, an adult who was known to the child acclimated the child to the lab via toy-play and was present in the room at all times. She (it was usually a woman) was seated behind a cardboard screen out of the direct sightlines of the subject to minimize any influence she might have on the child's behavior. Finally, one additional technical innovation was added: Bijou's child study laboratory was motorized!

By the mid-1950s, Bijou was convinced that the controlled environment of the human-sized Skinner box was an ideal place to conduct laboratory studies with children. Results seemed promising, and the technique was efficient. He designed the lab to be as close to the naturalistic setting of the classroom as possible, while preserving a high degree of experimental control. The only problem with a room-sized Skinner box was that children had to come to the room; the box was too big to move around. A solution soon presented itself. As Bijou wrote many years later, 'I was now convinced that laboratory studies with children should be conducted in controlled settings like infra-human animal studies. To augment the Institute facilities, I built a mobile laboratory, a converted house trailer, that could be easily towed to any nursery school in the Seattle area where additional studies could be carried out' (Bijou, 2001, p. 112). In addition to an efficient technique, Bijou now had a portable one.[22] To characterize Bijou's mobile laboratory as a Skinner box on wheels is not off the mark. As one behavioral psychologist and colleague of Bijou's wrote to Skinner in 1956, 'I'm due to teach summer school in Seattle, where Sid Bijou, you will be interested to know ... has an automobile trailer that is a Skinner-box for little kids.'[23]

Research and Service

In 1961, Bijou immersed himself in operant psychology, thus rounding out his conversion to the Skinnerian approach. He spent a sabbatical year at Harvard during which he audited Skinner's famous undergraduate lecture course 'Natural Science 114' and attended Pigeon Staff meetings which typically 'ended on a high note with a round of beer' (Bijou, 2001, p. 115). Meanwhile, his group at the ICD was experiencing its own series of high notes. As Todd Risley, one of the ICD's graduate student researchers, remarked of the convergence of people and projects at the Institute, '[T]he Institute of Child Development became caught up in a remarkable time of discovery and excitement ... People came from miles around to listen, to question, and to present their work' (Risley, 2001, p. 269).

Much of the excitement was fueled by an increasing number of demonstrations of the power of the operant approach in providing solutions to behavioral problems. Bijou's labs – both stationary and mobile – were supporting the research of a large group of graduate students and new faculty members, many of whom were quickly moving into applied areas. In 1962, Montrose Wolf, then a doctoral student at Arizona State University,[24] joined Sidney Bijou at the ICD. Wolf's task was to help head up a grant-funded human learning laboratory at Rainier State School for the developmentally disabled just outside of Seattle. Although Wolf was hired to run a human operant laboratory, his training and orientation predisposed him towards applied work. With colleagues at Arizona State, he had already helped design a token economy system to teach reading to preschool children (Staats, Staats, Schultz, and Wolf, 1962). Wolf was aware of the pioneering nature of application at this time, later noting:

> Few had made the leap from the lab to the other side of the one-way mirror or to schools or to homes. In fact, some were of the opinion that such a leap was premature and unwise because we didn't know enough, that we needed to wait for more basic human operant research. (Wolf, 2001, p. 290)

Regardless, Wolf seized the opportunities at Rainier to further develop applied behavioral techniques. The result was a combination of research and application.

Within two weeks of arriving at the University of Washington, Wolf was called into Bijou's office along with graduate student Todd Risley. Bijou had been contacted by the director of a nearby children's psychiatric hospital to consult on the difficult case of a severely autistic child who refused to wear his glasses. The child, christened Dicky in subsequent research reports, had recently had a cataract operation. He was required to wear glasses or face blindness within six months. Despite a three-month hospitalization, no one had been able to get him to wear his glasses. Bijou put Wolf and Risley on the case, and the result was their classic study with Dicky, who not only learned to wear his glasses, but went on to graduate from high school (Wolf, Risley, Johnston, Harris, and Allen, 1967; Wolf, Risley, and Mees, 1964; Wolf, 2001). As Risley retrospectively remarked, 'Mont never did the job he was hired to do – generate useful knowledge from a human-operant laboratory – but with the excitement and productivity of everything else, no one seemed to notice' (Risley, 2005, unpublished manuscript). Interestingly, Bijou credited his exposure to Ferster's work at Indiana for his willingness to take on the case in the first place. As he later noted, 'If it hadn't been for Charlie's program on autistic children, which I had visited several times, I don't know that we'd have dared to arrange a program with a severely disturbed child like Dicky' (Bijou, in Krasner, 1977, p. 593).

Clearly bitten by the bug of application, Montrose Wolf then collaborated with teachers at the ICD nursery school to help eliminate the regressive crawling of a three-year-old girl (Harris, Johnston, Kelley, and Wolf, 1964), and to increase the peer interactions of a severely isolate preschool girl, Ann (Allen, Hart, Buell, Harris, and Wolf, 1964). As Eileen Allen, the lead author on this latter report noted:

> Teachers learned to gather their own data (I coined the phrase *collecting data on the hoof*). We demonstrated that teachers could collect data that were the core of sound intervention programs for individual children and were also reliable to a high degree when matched with the data of independent reliability raters.[25]

In recalling the transition from basic research to applied research in this period, Bijou made explicit the link between the human operant labs and the study of children's behavior in natural settings: 'The methodology for studying children's behavior in natural settings was an expansion and adaptation of the laboratory operant conditioning method. It developed with the ... study in which the regressive crawling of a preschool girl was quickly eliminated' (Bijou, 2001, p. 117). The techniques of measurement and recording made their way from the room-sized Skinner box to the actual classroom. In doing so, however, they underwent certain necessary transformations. Continuous recording via pre-programmed equipment gave way to direct behavioral observation by trained observers. The reversal baseline design, involving (1) a baseline measurement of behavior, (2) introduction of a behavioral intervention, followed by (3) its removal (to see if behavior reverted to its baseline level), was used to ensure that the intervention (withdrawal of attention for undesirable behavior and systematic positive reinforcement of desirable behavior) was solely responsible for the behavior change. This was research *and* practice. As Allen and her colleagues wrote at the end of their report on Ann, 'Such a combination of the functions of research and service seems both practical and desirable' (Allen, Hart, Buell, Harris, and Wolf, 1964, p. 518). Many others agreed.

Deconstructing the Box

By the early 1960s, a body of work that employed Skinner's experimental methodology with humans – as well as other species – was well established. Although this research was undertaken primarily for the purpose of extending and testing the free operant method itself, it often held implications for application. Indeed, in this same very early period, the application of Skinnerian principles to individual behavior problems had already begun and was quickly taking hold of the field. The research from the human operant labs was not as impressive to those Skinnerians who were already using operant principles outside the box. Jack Michael,

Wolf's mentor and one of these Skinnerian pioneers, commented retrospectively that 'the idea that we were going to have to do research to prove that reinforcement works you know, that didn't seem plausible anymore, [it was] like gravity' (Michael, 2004, interview with the author).

To many Skinnerians, the efficacy of positive reinforcement and the power of shaping were face-evident. Tightly controlled replications of various reinforcement schedules with goldfish, dogs, chimps, young children, and schizophrenics, although interesting from a technical and scientific standpoint, seemed unnecessary as justification for actually *using* the techniques to pragmatic ends. As early as 1949, Paul Fuller had used operant procedures in a clinical setting to shape the arm movements of a 'vegetative human organism' (Fuller, 1949). Fuller's study became one of the classic 'firsts' in behavior modification, leading Sidney Bijou to remark to him years later, 'Paul, I don't know of anybody who got so much mileage out of one measly experiment!'[26]

In the late 1950s, a group of graduate students, including Montrose Wolf, began meeting at the University of Houston under the tutelage of Jack Michael. Michael, who was trained as a quantitative, experimental psychologist, had bought a copy of Skinner's *Science and Human Behavior* years earlier for a course he subsequently dropped, and it sat on his shelf for a while gathering dust (Michael, 2003). When he decided he needed more material for a course on learning he was about to teach, he finally cracked it open and was immediately drawn to the practical issues it addressed. In his words:

> When I try to think about why it was so attractive, it was the many realistic examples. I mean every page has something that illustrates the principle that Skinner had introduced in the early parts of the book. He illustrates the principle maybe by talking about pigeons, and then gives many everyday examples of the same phenomena in terms of normal, adult humans. (Michael, 2004, interview with the author)

For Michael, Skinner's jump from pigeons to humans was precisely the key to his appeal. Michael quickly assembled a group of students who were similarly interested in Skinner's ideas, and they set out to apply some of his principles to the problems they found in their own backyard – the university campus. Teodoro Ayllon, a member of the group and an existential psychologist by training, recalled being somewhat skeptical at first:

> Well, let me see, it really didn't grab me ... exactly. I was introduced to it by Jack Michael in the context of a course he was teaching but I couldn't

understand him too well, it was very hard reading for me to do. What I understood better was the emphasis on having a few subjects and intensive observation rather than loads of subjects and having to work out the statistics ... but I did not think necessarily, frankly, that it would work with people. (Ayllon, 2005, interview with the author)

Conversely, another member of the group, John Mabry, recalled the excitement of taking Skinner's principles from the classroom and applying them in his personal life. Faced with the challenges of raising an active two-and-a-half-year-old daughter, he self-consciously used reinforcement of incompatible behaviors to ensure that she would not venture onto a busy street near their home. He remarked, 'It was the first time that any course work in psychology, or any reading, had even suggested a clear application. Commonplace now (among a small segment of the population), this was intensely exciting then' (Mabry, 1996, p. 111).

Other examples could be invoked to demonstrate the development of applied research in this period of the late 1950s and early 1960s. As I have already mentioned above, Montrose Wolf's work and influence was an important part of this transition. As behavior analysts demonstrated the efficacy of their techniques on a patient-by-patient, child-by-child, or student-by-student basis, the momentum of application grew. Findings from human-sized Skinner boxes held little interest for this new breed of behavior shaper. As Risley later wrote of his mentor Wolf's attitude towards the work coming out of the human operant labs:

Wolf came to consider laboratory research on human behavior to be mostly a 'dead end in scientific trappings' and five years later when he created the editorial policy of the new *Journal of Applied Behavior Analysis,* he explicitly excluded laboratory purported-analogues, in favor of the in-context observation and investigation of real-world phenomena. (Risley, 2005, unpublished manuscript)

The lack of interest may have been mutual. Researchers trained in the spirit of the Pigeon Lab also viewed the work of their more pragmatic colleagues somewhat skeptically. As Jack Michael put it:

At that time, Lindsley and many of the operant conditioning people were very strongly methodologically oriented to the point where [they felt] you could not possibly collect reasonable data unless it was automatically

collected ... He was derogatory towards the kinds of things I would talk to
him about ... like the token economy, getting the kids to read and working
with various problems – he was not convinced that our report of what we
were doing was valid. (Michael, 2004, interview with the author)

For his part, Michael reported that human free operant research held
little appeal for him personally, although he respected Lindsley's work
and was glad he was doing it. Michael's group went full steam ahead
with application. When asked his opinion of the applied research of that
period, Lindsley remarked that he objected to it because it ignored rate
of response. But he also noted significant resistance to basic human
research and, belying his own biases, cited as an example the lack of
research on children raised in air cribs: 'It amazed me that 250 children
had been reared in air cribs, that's the Skinner baby box, whatever you
want to call it, and no one had put in a lever. No one had put in a lever'
(Lindsley, 2004, interview with author).

Bijou represented a more truly transitional figure. He was convinced of
the importance of experimental child research and devoted to it in his own
career, but he nonetheless facilitated the work of Wolf, Risley, and others
who exemplified the new breed of behavior modifier. As Michael noted:

I was aware of Bijou's work, and again Bijou and Baer were doing essentially research, experimental research on children's behavior. They were
not attempting to change behavior for practical purposes, they were not.
They were studying the behavior, just like Og Lindsley was studying it, and
it took Mont Wolf coming to Seattle, working with Sid for a while, to actually institute all of the modification stuff ... So Mont at Seattle was simply
starting behavior modification. Baer and Bijou were more uptight about
the methodological aspects of it. Mont wanted to get the girl to stop crawling. (Michael, 2004, interview with the author)

Application soon more or less monopolized the field, although the
distinction between research and application was often blurry as the
commonly used term 'applied research' demonstrated. Fairly rapidly,
a further deconstruction of the human Skinner box occurred: interventions with individual students in individual classrooms gave way to
the design of entire schools offering Skinnerian programs. Hospitals
and prisons also became hotbeds of contingency management. In
1968, Ayllon and colleague Nathan Azrin published their full-length

monograph describing a token economy program on a psychiatric ward. This program, and others like it, inspired a veritable explosion of behavior modification in institutions. The Skinner box was being gradually expanded in favor of total environments for the remediation of problem behaviors. It is to these total environments that I now turn, starting with the psychiatric ward.

chapter 3

Conditioning a Cure: Behavior Modification in the Mental Institution

To the uninitiated, behavior modification sounds complicated and dangerous. In this age of consumer rebellion, mental hospitals ... might well do without controversial programs. However, the hospitals need the magic of the new approaches, and perhaps they can be forgiven for jumping on bandwagons. The behavior modification bandwagon seems more substantial than most, as it is braced by concepts from research in the psychology of learning.

Martin, 1972, p. 287

Although the pharmacological revolution of the 1950s and the Community Mental Health and Patients' Rights movements of the 1960s brought some profound changes to service provision for the severely mentally ill, only in some cases were these improvements (see Barton and Sanborn, 1977; Stockdill, 2005). Moreover, they did not eradicate the phenomenon of the 'back ward psychotic' – the chronically institutionalized schizophrenic patient for whom neither drug regimens nor community support provided viable alternatives to full-time, in-patient care. As the above quote reveals, by the late 1960s psychiatry and psychology were still in search of effective ways to treat those patients whose plight seemed most hopeless. Psychoanalytic talking cures were among the only other tools in the psychiatrist's toolbox, and these too proved largely ineffective in revealing the roots of psychosis and returning the schizophrenic to reality. The question of how to move beyond palliative care and actually improve the functioning of the chronically mentally ill, many of whom had spent the better part of their lives in institutions, remained unanswered. Could Skinnerian psychologists provide a solution?

As I have shown in the previous chapter, by the early 1960s several groups of Skinnerian psychologists stood on the brink of full-scale application and were looking for problems to solve with their new technology. No human behavior problem seemed too difficult to tackle, not even the back ward psychotic. In the case of psychosis, however, Skinnerians brought not only a technological solution, but a reformulation of the problem. Psychosis should be treated as nothing more than psychotic behavior. With their goal of decreasing psychotic behavior itself, rather than understanding its etiology, along with a kit bag full of behavioral techniques to accomplish this goal, practitioners of behavior modification offered, if not magic, at least a common-sense, can-do approach to treating psychiatry's most challenging cases.

One of the most widespread applications of behavior modification in the mental hospital – and elsewhere – during the mid-to-late 1960s and early 1970s took the form of the token economy. Although tokens themselves – literally, plastic chips, coins, and cards, among other trinkets – had already been employed as generalized reinforcers to change individual behavior on a case-by-case basis by the early 1960s (and reports of these studies had been made in several published articles; e.g., Ferster and DeMyer, 1961), the first comprehensive token *economy* was developed and implemented by Teodoro Ayllon and Nathan Azrin at Anna State Hospital in Illinois between 1961 and 1967.

In the history of psychiatry, Ayllon and Azrin's 1968 monograph describing their token economy system for chronically institutionalized schizophrenics stands as a classic in the literature (Ayllon and Azrin, 1968). At Anna State, Ayllon and Azrin broke new ground in behavioral treatment by conceptualizing mental illness in purely functional, behavioral terms, and by designing a comprehensive token economy involving the entire staff and population of patients on a special ward. Unlike the largely psychoanalytic psychiatrists who ran most of the treatment programs in state hospitals and who saw behavioral aberrations as symptoms of deep-seated psychic conflict, Ayllon and Azrin chose to regard these 'symptoms' simply as behaviors like any others. In their formulation, if you could decrease or remove the aberrant behaviors and increase or shape socially acceptable ones, the patient would come close to resembling a non-psychotic individual. If the staff of a whole ward of patients could be taught to systematically award tokens for functional behavior, and patients could learn that these tokens could purchase a range of desirable commodities, behavior modification might prove its worth in the psychiatric hospital.

As word of Ayllon and Azrin's work spread, particularly after the publication of their interim report on activities at Anna State in 1965 (Ayllon and Azrin, 1965), a veritable explosion of token economies in classrooms, psychiatric wards, homes for the mentally retarded, reform schools, and prisons ensued. In this chapter, I document the prehistory of the Anna State token economy in the work of Teodoro Ayllon, and then describe Ayllon and Azrin's classic program in more detail. I then briefly outline the proliferation of the token economy in a variety of settings, including the mental hospital, but also in homes for children and adults with developmental disabilities, and in education. The late 1960s and early 1970s marked the heyday of the token economy as an institutional treatment approach. However, as I will note briefly at the end of this chapter and then document more fully in chapter 4, a number of practical, ethical, political, and legal issues curtailed the continuation of many programs and slowed the momentum of the token economy by the end of the 1970s.

Teodoro Ayllon and the Prehistory of the Token Economy

Teodoro Ayllon, a Bolivian-born, existentially trained clinician, arrived at the University of Houston in 1957. That same year, his soon-to-be mentor, Jack Michael, arrived as a faculty member and attracted a bevy of students interested in Skinner's ideas and how to apply them to human problems. Ayllon had actually come to work on his doctorate with Lee Meyerson, a rehabilitation psychologist with no a priori allegiance to Skinner's approach, although he too would come to appreciate its practical applications in his own field (see Meyerson, Kerr, and Michael, 1967). Ayllon, in fact, had little interest in operant psychology, despite Michael's enthusiasm, and remained somewhat skeptical of its apparent theoretical simplicity. Nonetheless, as Michael noted, Ayllon was eventually drawn to the Skinnerian approach because existential psychology was 'good at understanding but not doing,' and Ayllon was 'open to the idea of doing something practical – we could make things work with people – he liked that' (Michael, 2004, interview with author). And so Ayllon was attracted to Michael's group and soon joined them in discussing how to apply the principles of operant psychology to everyday problems.

As I alluded to in the previous chapter, the campus preschool at the University of Houston provided one of the first behavior-change projects that the group undertook. Interested in testing out the practical worth of behavioral principles, Ayllon approached the teachers at the preschool and asked them if they could identify any behaviors in the children that they might like to see changed. The only problem the teachers could come up with was that they had a little girl who did not like to color in her coloring book. Apparently, this unwillingness to color caused some disturbance, as coloring was a frequently invoked activity in the preschool and she would consistently cry and tantrum when asked to do so. So, taking the teachers' concern at face value and eager to try out operant theory in the 'real world,' Ayllon began to sit with the girl during coloring time, and whenever she turned her gaze towards the coloring book, he would deposit a small candy in her cup. Gradually, he proceeded to reinforce closer and closer contact with the coloring materials. Michael remarked that it took Ayllon about a couple of weeks to get the little girl coloring happily without a tantrum (Michael, 2004, interview with the author). This early success was quite gratifying to the young researchers. It seemed they had a technology that was relatively straightforward to implement and apparently highly effective. If this behavior could be shaped, what about others?

The next project the group undertook involved students attending a remedial summer reading course offered at a nearby high school. Students who needed help in reading before progressing from junior high to high school had to enrol in a course that required them to work through a series of reading workbooks. Pat Cork, one of the members of Michael's group, had a friend who was a teacher at the school. Again, the group inquired if there were any problems of human behavior that aspiring behavioral engineers could tackle. Apparently, some of the students were not working in their workbooks as instructed. The research group, assuming that the workbooks were in fact effective in teaching reading skills, decided to give the students points for correct answers in the workbooks.

Because these students were older than the children in the university preschool and had more diverse interests, the researchers decided to use points as generalized reinforcers which could be accumulated and used at the end of every class to buy small toys and trinkets, according to each student's desires. These points, which performed like money, were among the first tokens used in a behavior analytic program of behavior change.[1] Michael pointed out the similarity of this system to the system of monetary allowances that the children were used to and remarked that it was just a natural extension – a common-sense idea – that led them to use a points system. The program was never written up or published, and the researchers learned that although they could use token reinforcement to get the students to finish their workbooks, the students were not necessarily learning how to read effectively. Thus, setting an appropriate and relevant behavioral end goal was clearly key. Deciding on appropriate behavioral goals would prove, in fact, a recurring and rather thorny problem for the behavioral engineer.

The next step for Ayllon was an internship at Saskatchewan Hospital, a psychiatric hospital in Weyburn, Saskatchewan. Still a graduate student, Ayllon was in need of summer work and had a connection with one of the supervisors at the hospital. When he arrived at Saskatchewan, he was basically given free rein to try out operant principles on some of the hospitalized psychotic patients. Yet, Ayllon was skeptical:

> When I went to Saskatchewan what I had really in mind was a test for myself, it was a kind of a test that couldn't work ... I didn't think it [operant reinforcement] was going to work ... My view was, if I work with people [with whom] everybody's tried everything – including drugs – and it's only three months (I mean, I'm obviously not in the guild yet, I'm just a graduate student), I would try it for myself to see and show that perhaps this is really interesting. But I didn't see how it could work. You didn't know the people, and whatever they did was so far out that I didn't see how you could change them. (Ayllon, 2005, interview with author)

Thus, armed with a skeptical but enterprising attitude and access to the back wards, Ayllon quickly observed that the professionals most intimately involved in the day-to-day care of the patients were the psychiatric nurses. He quickly enlisted the help of the nurses in identifying which patient behaviors to change and in setting up and implementing individualized programs for a number of patients. In deciding which behaviors to modify, the nurses tended to identify the behaviors which were most disruptive in the day-to-day running of the ward and those which affected the safety of the patients and workers. For example, Lucille made frequent visits to the nursing station and disrupted and interrupted the nurses. Another patient's 'psychotic talk' was identified as problematic, since it often resulted in her being attacked by other patients. Another patient was physically assaultive, another refused to eat, and others exhibited hoarding behaviors. In each case, Ayllon analyzed the contingencies that seemed to maintain the behaviors (often the attention of the ward staff), and taught the nurses a variety of operant procedures to rearrange these contingencies, reduce the frequency of undesirable behaviors, and, in some cases, increase desirable behaviors.

In assessing the significance of this work, which resulted in a now classic article by Ayllon and Michael entitled 'The Psychiatric Nurse as a Behavioral Engineer' (Ayllon and Michael, 1959), Michael remarked, 'The fact was, it did not have much practical significance, except for making the lives of the nurses better ... But it did have theoretical significance – the psychotic individual was susceptible to the same reinforcers as normals – this was important' (Michael, 2004, interview with author).[2] Importantly, it also gave Ayllon valuable experience working with staff and patients in a ward environment, and convinced him that the operant approach could really work.

Ayllon returned to Houston after his summer in Weyburn and graduated with his PhD from the University of Houston in 1959. He was then hired back to the Saskatchewan Hospital for two postdoctoral years to continue his work with patients, supported by a grant from the Commonwealth Fund. In his second year at Weyburn, he was joined by Eric Haughton, with whom he explored the use of food as a reinforcer to control psychotic behavior (Ayllon and Haughton, 1962). With Haughton's technical expertise and the influence of Nathan Azrin and Ogden Lindsley's published article on the reinforcement of cooperative behavior (Azrin and Lindsley, 1956), Ayllon devised ever more elaborate systems to engineer behavior. For example, he attempted to set up a situation in which pairs of Weyburn schizophrenics would cooperate in pushing a sequence of buttons in order to receive a coin or penny which could then be used to gain access to a television set. His main objective was to show that the patients' behavior could become organized without the need for verbal instructions or communication, and that the penny itself appeared to have some value to the patient (Ayllon, 2005, interview with the author). Through this work, he convinced himself that even non-verbal patients could grasp the function and value of a generalized reinforcer.

When his two years in Saskatchewan came to a close, Ayllon once again began looking for work. Although applied behavior analysis, or applied behavior research as it was still being called, was intensifying on the west coast with Bijou's group in Washington, Ayllon was impressed with behavior analyst Nathan Azrin's published research, his methodological innovations, and his writing style. Reports of dark and damp Washington weather were also unappealing to the Bolivian-born Ayllon, and he began to cast about elsewhere for job opportunities. With the intercession of Israel Goldiamond, Ayllon made Azrin's acquaintance and Azrin invited Ayllon to join him in Illinois.

Azrin had graduated from Harvard in 1956 and was working as research director in the Illinois Department of Mental Health. It would prove to be a fateful pairing. Together, they began to conceptualize the Anna State token economy early in 1961. They received a grant to support the work in June of that year, and began implementation in November. Armed with extensive familiarity with the Skinnerian corpus, and direct experience working with both normals and hospitalized psychotics, Ayllon and Azrin set out to design a complete ward environment based on operant reinforcement theory.

The Anna State Token Economy

A state mental hospital is a severe testing ground for any theory of human behavior. Almost every conceivable behavioral difficulty can be seen there, often in its most extreme form ... Any simple answer that one might consider for the problems of one patient seem irrelevant for other patients ... It seems that every type of explanation has already been proposed, applied, and found wanting in its general application, including psychotherapy, group dynamics, recreation therapy, vocational therapy, drug therapy, etc. One feels compelled to do something – anything – to assist this forsaken segment of humanity. (Ayllon and Azrin, 1968, p. 1)

At Anna State, the segment of humanity to whom Ayllon and Azrin devoted a total of about six years was a group of forty-five female patients transferred into their 'special ward environment' on a rotating basis. That is, at any one time there were a maximum of forty-five patients on the special ward. In making their patient selection, Ayllon and Azrin specifically asked for the involvement of those patients who were benefitting the least – that is, not at all – from existing ward procedures elsewhere in the hospital. Supervisors were asked to identify the patients whom they would most like to transfer out of their own wards. Ayllon and Azrin described the women who came to them as disheveled, unkempt, and largely unintelligible or mute. They typically received only rare visits from family and friends (on average two visits a year), had come from rural environments, and had spent an average of sixteen years in the psychiatric institution. To describe them as forsaken didn't seem too far off the mark.

But what did this select group of women find on their new, special ward? In terms of physical specifications, the ward itself consisted of five patient dormitories, a kitchen and dining room, a recreation room with a token-operated television set, a nurse's station, an examining room, and two offices and a rest room for staff. On duty were a physician, a nurse, a psychologist, and the attendants. An average of two attendants worked the ward during the day, with one attendant staffing the night shift. Given that a typical psychiatric ward in this period might have one attendant for every hundred patients, it seemed that the special ward was indeed an improvement over standard operating procedure.

Once transferred to the 'motivating environment,' as Ayllon and Azrin christened their unit, patients were expected to choose an off-ward job as well as participate in on-ward duties in order to earn tokens that could be exchanged for a variety of reinforcers. In operant terms, these jobs were the 'responses.' In Ayllon and Azrin's formulation, serving meals, cleaning floors, and sorting laundry were responses that were defined as 'necessary' or 'useful' to the patient to function in the hospital environment (Ayllon and Azrin, 1965, p. 357). While this point would actually come under legal scrutiny later in the history of the token economy, their rationale was to engage the patients in functional and adaptive work activities that would assist in the day-to-day running of the hospital and the ward. They remarked that these kinds of work resembled the jobs that might be expected of the patients in the outside world, but noted that outside employment was not the end goal of the program, a point to which I will return.

The off-ward jobs that were offered to the patients included dietary worker (serving meals and cleaning tables), clerical worker (typing, answering the telephone), laboratory assistant (cleaning cages and floors in laboratory, filling water bottles), and laundry worker (feeding sheets and towels through mangle, folding linens). On-ward duties included helping run the kitchen and dining room, waitressing at meal times, providing secretarial assistance, cleaning the ward, serving as assistant janitor, laundry assistant, or nursing assistant, helping staff carry out grooming and recreational activities, running errands, and giving tours of the ward to visitors.

In addition to performing these duties, patients could also earn tokens by engaging in a number of self-care activities such as grooming, bathing, toothbrushing, exercising, and bed-making. The overarching philosophy was to provide a system in which the opportunity to engage in a whole range and variety of functional behaviors was maximized and every functional behavior was reinforced. Eliminating or decreasing dysfunctional behaviors that continued to interfere with an individual's ability to participate in the token economy was a secondary goal. As Ayllon and Azrin

(1968) stated, 'Full-time and active involvement of the patients in many and varied and useful activities was the objective of the program' (p. 24). In many cases, as functional behavior increased, the behavioral problems or 'symptoms' of disorder subsided. In cases where this did not occur, Ayllon and Azrin worked with individual patients to shape necessary behavior, such as self-feeding in the case of Wilma M., or to reduce maladaptive behavior, such as wearing excessive amounts of clothing, as in the case of Rita O.

Once earned, what would tokens buy the industrious psychiatric patient in the motivating environment? Ayllon and Azrin developed six categories of reinforcers: (1) privacy (for example, the opportunity to select a room in the dormitory, purchase a screen or room divider, or procure a personal cabinet); (2) leave from the ward, including walks on the hospital grounds and trips to town; (3) social interaction with staff, including private audiences with a variety of ward staff, chaplains, and social workers; (4) devotional opportunities, such as the option to attend religious services; (5) recreational opportunities, such as watching movies, the use of a radio, the choice of a television program; and (6) purchase of a wide variety of commissary items. Their rationale, simply put, was that in providing a wide range of reinforcers, they could provide something that would appeal to everyone.

Over the six years of the program, a total of 65 patients participated in the token economy. In their 1968 monograph, they reported that of these 65 patients, 58 performed at least some of the duties contributing to the functioning of the ward, defined as at least one hour of work per day for a minimum of forty days. Only seven patients failed ever to reach this level of work. In terms of these duties, 30 patients held one or more of the ward positions for over one year, and 10 held various positions for as long as three years. In the case of off-ward jobs, 20 of the 65 patients held one or more of these positions for one year or more, working six hours a day. Ayllon and Azrin concluded: 'The degree of useful employment of a large number of patients over such an extended period of time is significant because all of the patients selected for study in the motivating environment had a long history of idleness' (Ayllon and Azrin, 1968, p. 55). Further, they suggested that the nature and arrangement of work and its reimbursement approximated, for these patients, most of the conditions of employment in the natural environment.

Notably, Ayllon and Azrin did not use the criterion of discharge into the community as a measure of the success of their motivational system, even though some of their patients were discharged from the hospital to the adjacent half-way house. As they aptly noted, many of their patients were of such an advanced age (over sixty-five), had spent so much of their lives in the institution, and no longer had any connections with family, friends, or a social support network to which they could return, that discharge as an outcome measure made little sense. The institution had truly become home for most of these patients. In terms of treatment evaluation, Ayllon and Azrin preferred to stick directly to assessing the extent to which patients were engaged in 'useful and functional behaviors' (Ayllon and Azrin, 1968, p. 26). The success of the Anna State program lay in the extent to which inactive patients became active, and function replaced dysfunction.

Impact of Anna State

Ayllon and Azrin's reports of their work prompted visits from many interested researchers and practitioners. Many of these people took what they observed at Anna State and set up token economies in their own institutions, many of which served very different populations (for a review of token economies implemented in a wide range of settings in the 1970s, see Kazdin, 1977). The token economy approach was extended to the behavior of children in nursery schools, the physically and mentally disabled in sheltered workshops, juvenile delinquents in correctional institutions, and developmentally delayed adults in institutions for the retarded.[3]

The classroom provided especially fertile ground for the development of token economies. In reviewing the use of token economies in education, Krasner and Krasner (1973) noted the seminal influence not only of Ayllon and Azrin's work, but also of Sidney Bijou's associate Jay Birnbrauer, who was using token reinforcement in classrooms for mentally retarded pupils by the mid-1960s (see, for example, Birnbrauer and Lawler, 1964). Another early example of the use of the token economy with the mentally retarded was Mimosa Cottage, set up by University of Kansas Bureau of Child Research workers in 1965. Mimosa Cottage was a residential program for educable mentally retarded girls that employed a token economy to reinforce personal grooming behaviors, occupational and academic skills, and social behaviors. Unlike the Anna State token economy, the goal of the Mimosa Cottage program was to return at least some of the higher-functioning girls to the community (see Lent, 1968). Krasner and Krasner credited O'Leary and Becker with first extending the use of the token economy to a large class of children with behavior problems in a public school setting (O'Leary and Becker, 1967).

In addition to the proliferation of token economies in these diverse settings, many practitioners working with the chronically mentally ill took Anna State as a direct inspiration for setting up token economies on their own psychiatric wards, and also set about evaluating them (e.g., Atthowe and Krasner, 1968; Gripp and Magaro, 1971; Kale, Zlutnick, and Hopkins, 1968; Schaefer and Martin, 1966). In a 1969 survey of token economy programs in Veterans Administration hospitals, 27 token economy programs in 20 different hospitals involving about 935 patients were reported (Stenger and Peck, 1970). Nor was the token economy a purely American phenomenon. A 1973 review of behavior modification in the United Kingdom revealed 16 token economy programs in psychiatric hospitals and hospitals for the mentally handicapped at that time (Hall, 1973). In Australia, Winkler (1970) implemented a token economy at Gladesville Psychiatric Hospital, a large facility in Sydney.

By the mid-1970s, it seemed as though multitudes were jumping on the token economy bandwagon and it was on its way to becoming a widely implemented treatment approach in the psychiatric hospital. The token economy appeared to offer, if not magic, at least a substantial improvement over custodial care and possibly a significant improvement over other forms of therapy. In fact, in 1977, amidst calls for more tightly controlled and rigorously designed studies comparing token economies to other interventions (Carlson, Hersen, and Eisler, 1972; Kazdin and Bootzin, 1972), Gordon Paul and Robert Lentz published just such a study. *Psychosocial Treatment of Chronic Mental Patients* was the culmination of a ten-year process in which they systematically compared three treatment approaches for the chronically institutionalized mental patient. As Paul wrote, 'The comparative project involved three ongoing groups of the most severely debilitated chronic mental patients ever subjected to systematic study' (Paul and Lentz, 1977, Preface). They randomly assigned 84 patients to three conditions: a milieu therapy program, a social learning therapy program, and usual hospital care. The same staff administered both the milieu and social learning programs. The primary component of the social learning program was a highly specific token economy involving structured educational activities. The milieu program consisted of living groups in which nine to ten patients per group were charged with exerting pressure on individual members to change by engaging in life skills or academic classes.

Paul and Lentz concluded, based on an extensive array of outcome measures as well as follow-up and aftercare data, that the patients who participated in the social learning group achieved greater discharge

rates, were maintained longer in the community, and required less psy-
chotropic medication than the patients in the other two groups. Certainly this was good news for the token economy. Or was it?

Decline of the Token Economy in the Psychiatric Hospital

Despite promising scientific evidence for the efficacy of token programs,
and their rapid proliferation in the 1970s, the number of psychiatric ward
token economies actually declined over the 1980s and 1990s, and are infre-
quently used today (see Dickerson, Tenhula, and Green-Paden, 2005, for a
contemporary assessment and review). As Glynn (1990) has noted:

> In writing about recent advances in token economy approaches in the treat-
> ment of schizophrenia and other serious psychiatric disorders, one faces a
> paradox. The token economy represents one of the most well-validated,
> comprehensive, nonmedical treatments for serious psychiatric illness, yet
> surveys indicate that it is currently rarely used in clinical settings. (P. 383)

In analyzing and explaining this perplexing decline, authors have
repeatedly noted a number of contributing factors internal to the
token economy, as well as the impact of developments external to it.
First, despite their effectiveness, token economies were not easy to set
up and implement. Ayllon and Azrin had near-perfect conditions at
Anna State. It was a small, innovative hospital organized into separate
departments, each of which was given a high degree of autonomy. The
researchers could make changes within the ward quickly and efficiently, with no need for concomitant institution-wide changes or
approval by institutional committees. They had the support of the
superintendent, and dealt with a small number of both patients and
staff, maximizing cooperation with and commitment to the program.
This also made it easier to train staff. Indeed, staff cooperation and
training emerged as a significant obstacle in many subsequent programs (see Hall and Baker, 1973, for a discussion of this and other
problems). Staff resistance was often rooted in the perception that
token economy programs were too much work, required too much
record-keeping, and were too regimented. Token economy programs,
specifically, were often tarred with the same brush as behavior modification generally: they were too mechanistic; they were punitive, inhumane; and they undermined the patient-clinician relationship. Token
economies, from the staff perspective, were not that much fun.

In addition to overcoming staff resistance, proponents of the token economy had to convince hospital administrators that the programs were worth the extra money and resources that they required. Not only did token economies require more staff and more staff time for training, implementation, and ongoing evaluation, they also required an increased budget for purchasing the supplies and reinforcers required to run the economy.

Combined with these internal factors were a number of changes in mental health policy during the period token economies were developed that created an inhospitable environment for any treatment program requiring long-term hospital stays. Glynn (1990) reported that from the 1950s to the 1970s, the average length of a hospital stay in a psychiatric institution dropped from six months to three weeks. Health insurance companies and government Medicaid and Medicare programs in the United States increasingly paid for only shorter stays, and even in state hospitals a revolving-door style of treatment took hold. This of course coincided with the increasing emphasis on community-based treatment for the seriously psychiatrically ill, making the implementation of token economies, which required a fairly high degree of environmental control and long in-patient stays, increasingly untenable.

Finally, as will be discussed in greater detail in the next chapter, several legal decisions in the 1970s pertaining to the treatment of the institutionalized mentally ill forced changes to, and restricted the purview of, the token economy. In 1972, the *Wyatt vs. Stickney* ruling dictated that institutionalized psychiatric patients have the right to basic amenities such as access to their personal property, a comfortable bed, a chair and bedside table, nutritious meals, flexible schedules for eating, bathing, and exercise, access to a recreation room with a television, and so on. This ruling eliminated many of the reinforcers that had been used to motivate behavior in the token economy. The court also concluded in this ruling that involuntary patient labor contributing to the operation or maintenance of the institution was not permissible, even if it were deemed therapeutic. Further, patients who volunteered to work could do so only if paid the minimum wage, and no other incentives, such as access to hospital grounds, day passes, etc., could be made contingent on such work. Finally, the doctrine of confinement in the least restrictive environment meant that treatment decisions had to be carefully justified, and patient movement within the hospital and outside of it could not be arbitrarily restricted, that is, on closed wards (for a detailed review of these and other legal issues pertaining to the token economy, see Kazdin, 1978, pp. 346–72).

It is fair to say that Ayllon and Azrin could not have implemented their program at Anna State in the form they did if they had arrived there ten years later. Although these rulings did not quash the token economy completely, they certainly demanded that administrators become more creative in designing their programs. They also contributed to the growing public perception that the token economy, at least as it was originally conceived, was inhumane and exploitative. But what of the patients themselves? Was there any indication that they found the motivating environment either an improvement or a burden?

In one of the only reports, if not *the* only report, of patient reaction to a token economy on a state hospital psychiatric ward, Douglas Biklen, then a doctoral student at the University of Michigan, outlined both his reactions and the reactions of patients to the enthusiastic attempts of two psychologists and their students to implement a token economy: 'In 1971, I spent nearly five months observing a behavior modification program in a locked state hospital ward for 53 so-called chronic schizophrenic women' (Biklen, 1976, p. 53). His period of participant-observation spanned twenty visits to the ward, during which time he interacted casually with patients, observed the efforts of the psychologists, students, and ward staff, and saw the token economy at work. Based on these observations, he highlighted a number of concerns. First, he questioned the objectivity of the program administrators in doling out tokens. The definitions of the behavioral goals to which patients were asked to aspire seemed vague at times, and the evaluations of whether they had achieved these goals appeared fairly subjective. For example, in the category 'General Behavior,' patients could be rated from 'bizarre' and 'obnoxious' to 'creative' and 'feminine' (p. 57), with their attendant point values. He opined that the token economy appeared to reinforce 'institutional' patient behaviors, that is, those that made the functioning of the ward and the institution easier. This often ended up infantilizing patients, as when they would earn stars for participating in the craft program, or for interacting with Santa when he made his annual holiday appearance on the ward. Biklen concluded:

> The professors, like their students, believed sincerely and intensely in the effectiveness of their enterprise. It seemed never to enter their thinking … that by rewarding patients with stars and cigarettes or by leading them in Christmas parties that more resembled parties of elementary school days (Santa came dressed in full attire), they were defining patients as 'child-like' and reinforcing an old institutional theme. The professors, far from seeing any dehumanization in their plans, saw themselves as change agents. (Biklen, 1976, p. 59)

But how did the patients respond? Did they, in fact, greet Santa with childlike glee? As one patient put it, 'I think this system stinks. They can go shove the whole thing as far as I'm concerned. I don't care about the stars.' Another patient confessed to Biklen, 'I had more privileges before this system started. They want me to mop floors and mop more floors. For what?' (p. 59). Based on these and other reactions, Biklen concluded that in fact many of the patients used strategies of subtle resistance, mockery, and anger to express their opposition to the token economy. Although stripped of institutional power, they nonetheless found ways to exert power over a system to which they were involuntarily subjected. For their part, the program administrators and students really did feel that in activating the patients, they were helping them.

This account highlights many of the problems that beset the token economy, especially as the legal rulings outlined above unfolded in the 1970s. Some creative research practitioners, convinced of the value of offering some form of effective treatment, were able to work within the parameters of these rulings and continued to carry the torch of the token economy. Although the Anna State program dissolved when Ayllon left to take a full-time academic appointment at Georgia State University and Azrin was no longer interested in overseeing it, programs like those at Camarillo State Hospital in California, which began in 1970, continue to this day.[4]

Conclusion

So what implications does this account of the prehistory and history of the token economy on the psychiatric ward have for our understanding of the development of applied behavior analysis? First, it seems that in its earliest stages, the use of operant procedures to change human behaviors was motivated by and undertaken with a confidence that the basic laws of behavior, established in the animal laboratories, would hold true even in these very different, and increasingly complex, environments. By and large, the problems initially chosen by these new behavioral engineers were circumscribed enough that this proved largely true, and there was a burst of enthusiasm as to what operant principles could accomplish in changing human behavior. There was also a general trend towards presenting these human behavior change ventures as applied experiments, combined with a willingness on the part of the basic research community to accept and publish this work. As applied researchers gained sophistication, programs of behavior change became experiments themselves, and rather elaborate ones at that. This was reflected in the development of A-B-A research designs, for example, in which an intervention would be implemented, removed, and implemented again to show that behavior change was the result of the intervention and not random factors. This was both experimentation and application rolled into one. However, the fact remained that the new applied behavior analysts were spreading their science from the laboratory into a whole new – and different – laboratory of life. This would, in turn, change the science itself.

As Skinner noted in his autobiography, 'People *were* [italics in original] different from rats or pigeons, but we should never know how different until we had studied them as we studied other species' (Skinner, 1983a, p. 54). It was in the late 1950s to early 1960s that Skinnerian psychology made its first conclusive steps beyond rat and pigeon psychology, providing the impetus for what would become, not only a science, but a *technology* of human behavior. With the rapid expansion of behavior modification into schools, prisons, and hospitals in the 1970s, many experimentalists became worried that their applied colleagues had lost sight of their basic science origins and were starting to run 'fast and loose' with a set of techniques that had not been experimentally tested or explored. Their call for closer links between the experimental and applied branches of behavior analysis continues to this day (see Sidman, 2004). Questions of how, why, under what circumstances, and with what exceptions, basic behavioral laws can be applied to human behavior, continue to fall under the behavior analysts' sphere of investigation.

Although coincidental, it is perhaps significant that 1968, the year Ayllon and Azrin published their monograph, was the same year that the *Journal of Applied Behavior Analysis* (*JABA*) began publication (see Laties and Mace, 1993, for an overview of the first twenty-five years of this journal). *JABA* had been preceded ten years earlier, in 1958, by the *Journal of the Experimental Analysis of Behavior* (*JEAB*). The decade between the foundings of these two journals – the first experimental, the later applied – was a pivotal one for the growth and extension of Skinner's principles beyond the laboratory. Their use in the psychiatric hospital, in the form of the token economy, was one example of this rapid extension from the laboratory to life. The reform school would soon provide another promising venue for the application of operant techniques. After visiting Ayllon and Azrin at their Anna State program, Harold Cohen envisioned, not a 'motivating environment' for his young charges, but a 'new learning environment,' as he and his colleague James Filipczak were to call their real-life experiment at the National Training School for Boys in Washington, DC (Cohen and Filipczak, 1971). Their new learning environment pushed the physical boundaries of the box, and the purview of the technology of behavior, even further.

chapter 4

Crime and Punishment:
Contingency Management in the Prison System

Now that Esquire has chosen both of us as among the 100 most important people in the world, I screw my courage to the point of writing you again. I recently attended a meeting of the Board of Directors of the Institution for Behavioral Research in Silver Spring, Maryland. Four years ago they began an experiment in the National Training School for Boys using a contingency-management design with serious juvenile delinquents ... The boys were on the program from three months to one year. They were then released from the school. A follow-up made three years later showed that the recidivism rate is about half what would otherwise be expected ... The state has saved the cost of the experiment many times over ... As one important man to another, shouldn't something be done?[1]

B.F. Skinner to McGeorge Bundy, 1970

In 1964, sixteen young inmates at the National Training School for Boys in Washington, DC, participated in an innovative pilot program designed to boost their academic achievement by placing them in a total learning environment. Named CASE I, or Contingencies Applicable to Special Education, it was spearheaded by Harold Cohen, an educator and environmental designer who had become convinced of the importance of the environment in influencing behavior, especially *learning* behavior. With his collaborator, James Filipczak, Cohen designed a pilot program involving a small sample of the National Training School's so-called juvenile delinquents. The pilot program ran for about eight months, from 24 February 1965, to 31 October 1965. It was followed by an expanded year-long program, CASE II, in which forty-one young men lived and studied together in a special building designed specifically to change and expand their academic and social repertoires.

The CASE II project became a template for prison programs across the United States in a period that saw a veritable explosion in the use of contingency management (a general term subsuming token economy approaches), not only in prisons, but also in schools, institutions for the mentally retarded, and psychiatric institutions (see previous chapter). Whereas the token economy offered back ward psychotics the possibility of effective treatment instead of custodial care, in prisons, contingency management revived the hope – at least briefly – that rehabilitation could serve as a reasonable goal of incarceration. In a penal system riddled with corruption and stressed beyond limit, in a society recovering from the civil unrest and urban riots of the 1960s, almost any attempt to 'treat' the problems of crime, violence, and delinquency received a hearing. It was this brief cultural opening that provided eager behavior analysts with an opportunity to try to make a difference in the penal system – a system traditionally designed to punish, rather than reward. Not everyone, however, regarded behavior modification as a hopeful development for prison reform and prisoner rehabilitation. As we shall see, for some it represented a coercive ploy to increase institutional control and deny prisoners their remaining rights.

Public scrutiny of behavior modification in prisons intensified in the early 1970s, and culminated in a House of Representatives oversight hearing on 27 February 1974 before the Subcommittee on Courts, Civil Liberties, and the Administration of Justice of the Committee on the Judiciary to evaluate behavior modification programs in the Federal Bureau of Prisons. By this time, behavior modification – referred to by some as methods of behavior control – had attracted national attention. The phrase 'behavior modification' had become an umbrella term for a panoply of interventions ranging from brainwashing, electric shock, and aversive conditioning, to rewards for good behavior. Controversy over research programs involving these procedures catalyzed a Senate Subcommittee investigation, entitled *Individual Rights and the Federal Role in Behavior Modification,* presented to Congress in November of 1974. Eventually, in combination with a number of other factors, concern over the use and misuse of behavior modification contributed to the formation of the National Commission for the Protection of Human Subjects of Biomedical and Behavioral Research (see Rutherford, 2006).

So how did CASE II, described by Skinner as 'landmark in penal reform' (Skinner, 1971b, p. xviii), contribute to setting this complex chain of events in motion? In the first part of this chapter, I outline Harold Cohen's pioneering project. As one of the earliest programs of its kind, it served as a prototype of what could be accomplished with the cooperation of prison administrators, adequate resources, and a captive population.[2] It also served as the inspiration for other programs of its kind as behavior analysts designed programs across the country. After outlining the CASE project, I examine two other programs designed by behavior analysts for adult inmates in the federal prison system and chart how the expansion of behavior modification in the prison milieu was cause for both optimism and alarm. Finally, I discuss the specific program that catalyzed much of this negative attention, and outline how professional psychology, the newly emerging profession of behavior analysis, and the federal government responded to these concerns.

A CASE in Point

Harold Cohen was perhaps an unlikely architect of a comprehensive token economy program for juvenile delinquents. As a former student of R. Buckminster Fuller at the Institute of Design in Chicago, Cohen was neither a direct student of Skinner nor a psychologist. However, he was an educator who was keenly interested in the influence of the physical environment on human behavior and human learning. Cohen was recruited from Chicago to Southern Illinois University (SIU), where he was charged with setting up a design school. Once there, he ended up designing a school.

Soon after arriving at SIU, Cohen met and was heavily influenced by a cadre of Skinnerian psychologists. Teodoro Ayllon and Nathan Azrin were there, and were setting up their token economy program at nearby Anna State Hospital. The outspoken Israel Goldiamond was also on faculty at the university. From these men Cohen learned about operant psychology and the power of the systematic use of positive reinforcement. He also observed Ayllon and Azrin's token economy at Anna State. Thus, when the president of the university approached Cohen with the dilemma of what to do with the large segment of the high school population who, although guaranteed a spot in the state university system, were literally not making the grade, Cohen took up the challenge of designing a total learning environment. With a class of about sixty-five students selected from the lower one-third of Illinois's graduating high school seniors, Cohen designed the 'Experimental Freshman Year' program, in which he attempted to boost the performance of the state's 'low-achievers.'

To achieve this daunting goal, he relied on his experience as a designer, the principles of Skinnerian psychology, and recent advances in programmed instruction. Interestingly, a key feature of his program was individual cubicles, which were essentially large cardboard booths providing a controlled environment for studying and learning. As Israel Goldiamond wrote of Cohen's work in a letter to Skinner:

> Harold has complete control of a class of 65 … students, chosen simply on the basis of recommendation from their principals that they were bright kids who simply didn't study. He keeps them the entire school day. Special booths have been constructed (out of cardboard for $7.50 wholesale: these are controlled environments for study) in which they do their studying. They are to do only school work there, and if they feel like doing something else, they leave; there are other behavioral devices for stimulus control of study behavior, including contingencies. The booths have a book case, a desk, a typewriter table, and a telephone; the staff calls the students and asks how they are doing; they can call for specific help. One student to a booth, incidentally. Since, if they do not study, they must leave the booth, we felt that such might constitute negative reinforcement. Accordingly, the room they can go to to escape study has a juke box which plays classical records, Shakespeare poems, closed circuit educational TV, and the like.[3]

In fact, Cohen set up the program on an unoccupied floor of a campus building. On this floor there were two lounges, a lecture room, an area for group work, and an area for the cubicles.[4] The cubicles were reserved for study only; if students wanted to engage in any other activities, they were free to do so by leaving the cubicles and going to the lounge. In this way, the cubicles became associated exclusively with study behavior, and contained everything the students might need to carry out this task, from periodic tables to typewriters.

Through his exposure to behavior analytic colleagues at SIU and his experience with the Experimental Freshman Year program, Cohen was converted to the Skinnerian approach and subsequently left SIU for a position at the recently founded Institute for Behavioral Research (IBR) in Silver Spring, Maryland. Charles Ferster was one of the first researchers at the IBR and served as its executive director during 1962–3. Many of the projects run under its auspices were educational and community-oriented. During his tenure there, Cohen was awarded grants from the Office of Juvenile Delinquency and Youth Development of the Department of Health, Education, and Welfare. With this grant support, he put his interest in education, his experience at SIU, and his knowledge of behavioral principles to work in designing the CASE programs.[5]

Cohen and his colleagues arrived at the National Training School (NTS) with an ambitious mandate: to take a random sample of NTS inmates from all grade levels, place them in a total learning environment, and, over the course of one year, prepare as many of them as possible either to be able to return to the public school system or pass a high school equivalency exam.[6] There were two key components of the program. The first was a token economy in which the students could earn points for academic performance. The second was the design of the physical environment itself, which was arranged to maximize academic achievement and provide numerous opportunities for reinforcement, from gaining entrance to the lounge to earning a private room.

The program participants were housed in a completely separate building on the NTS grounds – their own, elaborate, multi-level Skinner box. The building, Jefferson Hall, became Cohen's behavioral laboratory. He soon found it to be an ideal site for his research. As he put it:

When we first started CASE I, I was worried whether we could work in a 'penal institution.' I had preconceptions about prisons and what constituted a free or restricted environment. I soon learned what the medical profession had learned long before me – that the prison environment presents one of the finest laboratories for human research that is available for researchers in a free society. I soon realized that the university places more constraints on educational research than does the Federal Bureau of Prisons. (Cohen, 1968, p. 23)

Thus, under the fairly unrestrictive aegis of the Federal Bureau of Prisons, Cohen was able to randomly select forty-one participants for the program. Participation was not voluntary. The sample was racially mixed, although the white participants were largely from the southern United States and the black participants were largely from more northern states.[7] Most of the boys had dropped out of school before being committed to the NTS for a variety of crimes, including homicide, robbery, rape, and automobile theft. Once selected for the program, the boys were extensively evaluated and tested to ascertain their existing levels of academic ability across a variety of subjects. They then received individualized educational packages consisting of programmed courses, regular texts, and lecture classes. Participation in the academic program was voluntary, but the only way to earn points in the CASE program was by studying for an hourly wage[8] or getting 90 per cent or better on a test. Points earned could then be cashed in for a variety of different reinforcers. The behavioral goals of the program were operationalized as primarily educational, but as the program progressed, correctional officers were given the authority to award discretionary points for what they perceived as exceptionally good behavior in other areas. For example, one officer consistently reinforced students who made their beds and kept their rooms tidy. Another officer rewarded good language (Cohen and Filipczak, 1971, p. 13).

Once points were earned, the 'Student Educational Researchers,' as they were christened, could choose to spend them in a variety of ways. Popular choices included soft drinks, milk, potato chips, Polaroid snapshots, entrance to and time in the lounge or library, smoke breaks, rental of a private room, rental of books and magazines, purchase of private tutoring, and purchase of goods from a mail order catalogue. In effect, the inmates were paid to study and learn much like they would be paid for a regular job in the outside world.[9] Like ordinary citizens, they could choose not to study, but they would then receive no pay. The result was that they would have no money to buy the privileges that had been accorded them upon entry to the program, such as a private room.[10] They would be forced to go on 'relief status,' in which their living conditions reverted to the standard prison living conditions in the NTS. This meant little privacy, standard issue NTS clothing, standard prison meals, no visiting with friends in private rooms, no Sunday visitors except regular family, and enforced lights out.

Integral to the implementation of the program was the layout of Jefferson Hall itself. In their 1971 monograph, Cohen and Filipczak described the design of each floor and explained how each space was designed to function in a specific way. Access to certain parts of the building, such as the aforementioned lounge, was built into the token economy. Other parts of the building, such as the educational floor on the second level, were designated areas where certain behaviors were expected to take place. All students were constantly monitored and clocked in and out of certain areas designated by function. As a result, detailed data on the length of time each student spent in each area of the building were available to the researchers: 'The individual student was clocked in and out of each area ... This procedure provided an exact record for each individual over hundreds of calendar days, in terms of activities in functional locations and time measured in hundredths of an hour' (Cohen and Filipczak, 1971, p. 109). It was clear that one of the keys to the functioning of the program was being able to use physical space to influence and monitor the behavior of the program participants.

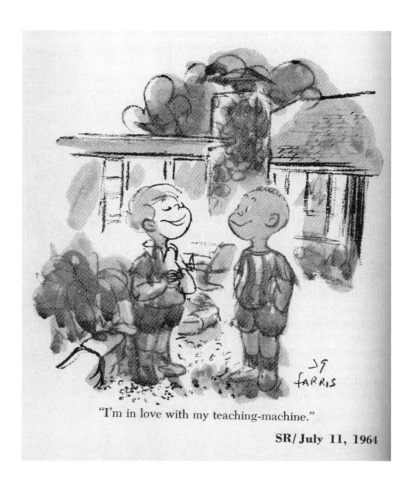

"I'm in love with my teaching-machine."

SR/July 11, 1964

This cartoon, which appeared in the 11 July 1964 issue of *Saturday Review*, makes reference to the then-ubiquitous teaching machine, prototypes of which were developed by B.F. Skinner and other inventors. The teaching machine was a centerpiece of the educational technology movement in the United States during the Cold War era. (*Saturday Review*)

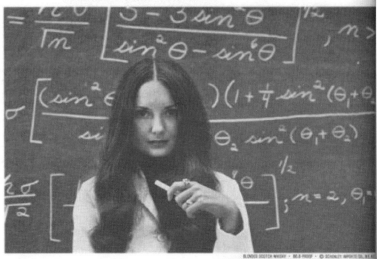
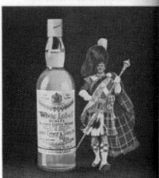
Sheila Ann T. Long, physicist, featured as part of a promotional campaign for Dewar's whiskey. Notice that she has listed Skinner's *Beyond Freedom and Dignity* as 'last book read.' (*Dewar's*)

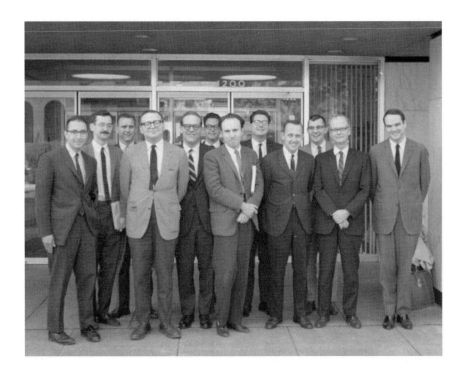

A group of behavior analysts at the Office of Economic Opportunity Conference on Applications of Operant Techniques to the Job Corps, held 19 and 20 May 1966. In the back row, from left to right, are John McKee, Jack Michael, Todd Risley, and David Lyon. In the middle row, from left to right, are Douglas Porter and Montrose Wolf. In the front row, from left to right, are Joel Wolfson, Israel Goldiamond, Harold Cohen (architect of the CASE program), Roger Ulrich, B.F. Skinner, and John Throne. Not shown, but attending the conference, were Charles Ferster, James Holland, and Lloyd Homme. (Courtesy of Harvard University Archives and Julie Vargas, HUG FP 60.90 p Box: Subject File ca 1932–1979 Folder 4 of 4)

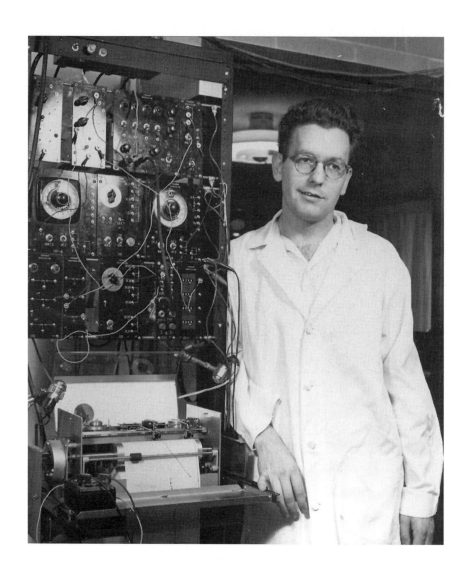

Jack L. Michael with his experimental apparatus at the University of Houston, 1957. (Courtesy of Jack L. Michael)

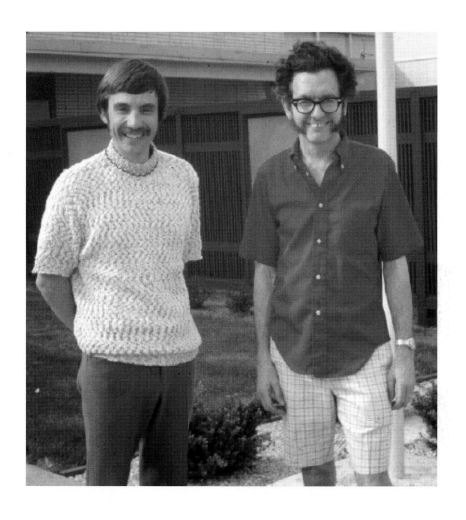

W. Scott Wood (left), organizer and participant in the 1974 Drake Conference on Professional Issues in Behavior Analysis, and Jack L. Michael, chair of the conference. They are pictured here in the late 1960s. (Courtesy of Jack L. Michael)

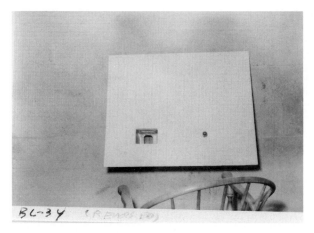

The wall-mounted console for research subjects in Ogden Lindsley's experiments at the Behavior Research Laboratory at Metropolitan State Hospital in the late 1950s and early 1960s. When the plunger manipulandum on the right was pulled, the subject would receive a reinforcer via a chute ending in the opening on the left. (Courtesy of Nancy Hughes Lindsley and the Ogden Lindsley Archive)

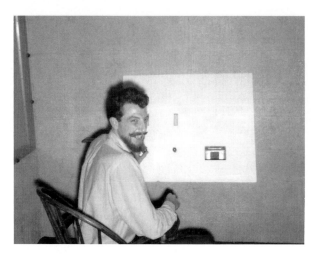

Ogden Lindsley, director of the Behavior Research Laboratory at Metropolitan State Hospital, in the late 1950s, in front of the apparatus he designed for the subjects in his room-sized Skinner boxes. (Courtesy of Nancy Hughes Lindsley and the Ogden Lindsley Archive)

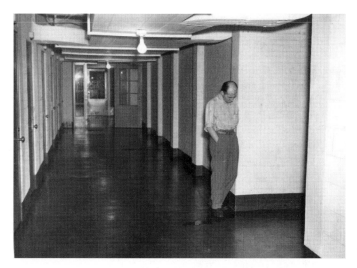

A patient with catatonic schizophrenia waiting in the corridor of Ogden Lindsley's Behavior Research Laboratory for his daily session in one of the experimental rooms (doors at left). (Courtesy of Nancy Hughes Lindsley and the
Ogden Lindsley Archive)

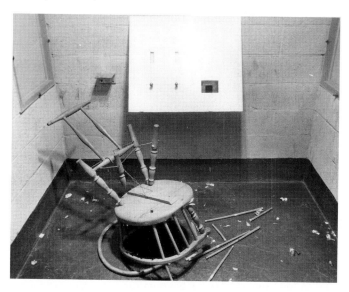

One of Ogden Lindsley's room-sized Skinner boxes in the aftermath of a violent
patient. (Courtesy of Nancy Hughes Lindsley and the Ogden Lindsley Archive)

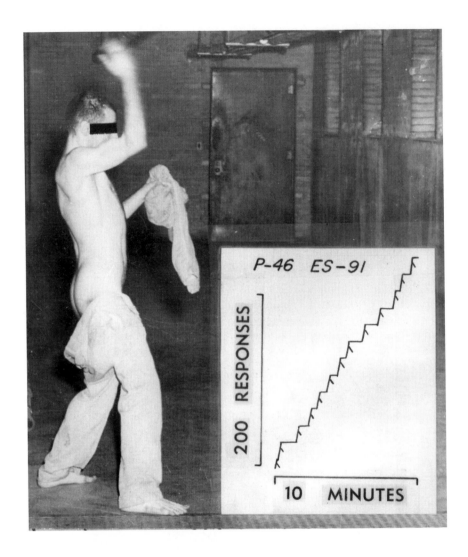

A schizophrenic patient on his way from his hospital ward to the Behavior Research Laboratory for his ninety-first experimental session. The chart at lower right shows the rate and pattern of his operant responses over a ten-minute period in the room-sized Skinner box. (Courtesy of Nancy Hughes Lindsley and the Ogden Lindsley Archive)

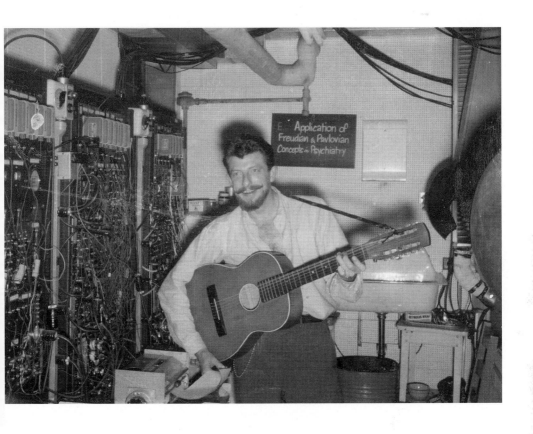

Ogden Lindsley playing his guitar in the control room at the Behavior Research Laboratory. (Courtesy of Nancy Hughes Lindsley and the Ogden Lindsley Archive)

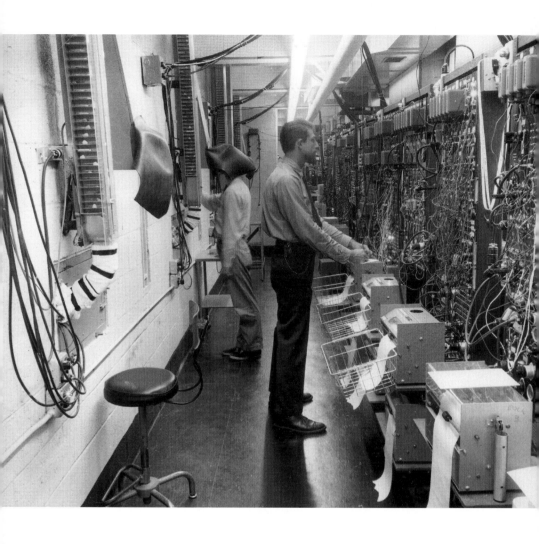

Ogden Lindsley overseeing the recording equipment in 'apparatus alley' behind the experimental rooms at the Behavior Research Laboratory. (Courtesy of Nancy Hughes Lindsley and the Ogden Lindsley Archive)

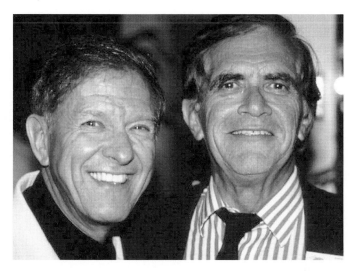

Teodoro Ayllon (left) and Nathan Azrin, who conceptualized and implemented the first token economy on a psychiatric ward at Anna State Hospital in the late 1960s. (Courtesy of Jack L. Michael)

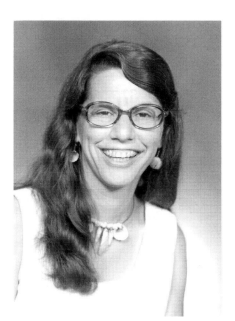

Stephanie B. Stolz, chair of the American Psychological Association Commission on Behavior Modification, pictured here around the time of the establishment of the commission in 1974. The commission investigated the uses and misuses of behavior modification and made recommendations regarding the regulation of behavioral techniques. (Courtesy of Stephanie B. Stolz)

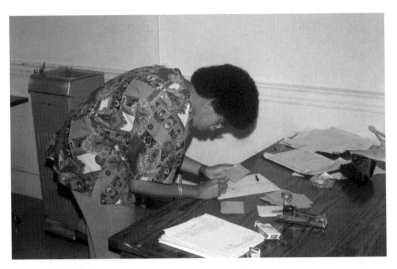

A research assistant recording data in the contingency management program designed and implemented by Scott Geller and his colleagues at Richmond State Penitentiary in 1974. (Courtesy of E. Scott Geller)

CMP CARD

NAME _Paul Hamlin_

WEEK OF _Sept. 1, 1974_

LAST WEEK EARNINGS _____

BALANCE _____00_____

A 'credit card' used to keep track of points earned by participants in the token economy designed by Scott Geller and colleagues.

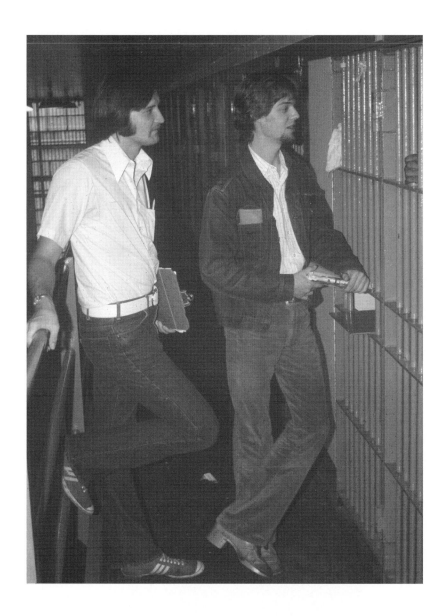

Two research assistants observing and recording an inmate's behavior in Scott Geller's contingency management program, Stage 1, at Richmond Penitentiary in Virginia in the early 1970s. (Courtesy of E. Scott Geller)

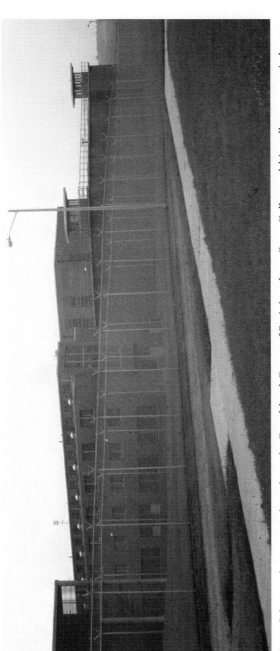

One of the maximum security prisons in Goochland County, Virginia, where Scott Geller and his colleagues carried out a stage in their contingency management program. (Courtesy of E. Scott Geller)

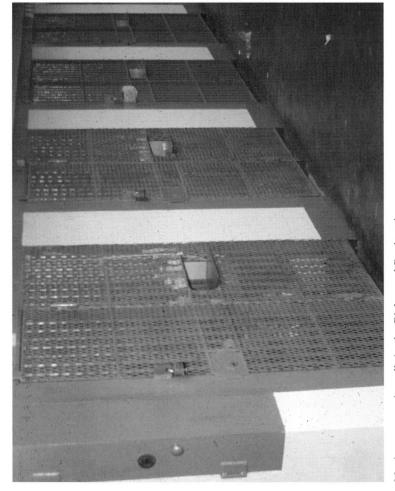

Maximum security cells in the Richmond Penitentiary.

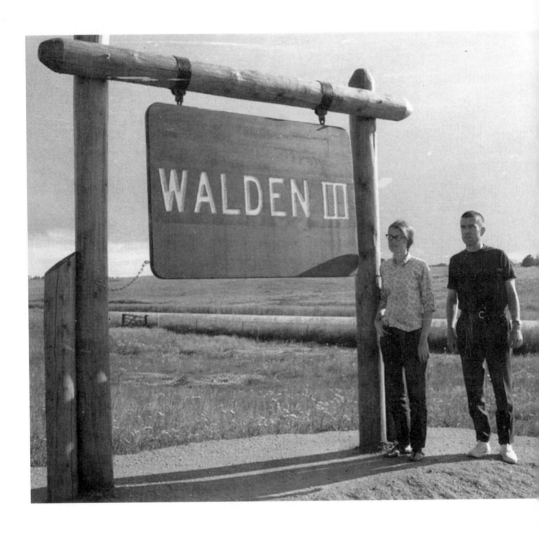

An unidentified man and woman standing in front of a sign for a Walden III community in Colorado Springs, Colorado, 1967. (Courtesy of Harvard University Archives and Julie Vargas, HUG FP 60.90 p Box: Subject File ca 1932–1979 Folder 1 of 4)

So what happened to the Student Educational Researchers? The main goal of the CASE program was to boost educational and academic achievement. Overall, according to its developers, it met this goal remarkably well. Participants' grade levels at the beginning of the program were measured across five subject areas – Reading, English, Science, Mathematics, and Social Studies. According to their entrance placement tests, none of the participants had reached either the junior or senior levels (encompassing grades 8–12) in any of these areas except Reading, where 37 per cent of participants were reading at the junior level (grades 8–10). By the time this group had completed the program, 26 per cent had achieved senior level status in Reading, 33 per cent had achieved senior level status in English, 18 per cent were seniors in Science, 25 per cent were seniors in Math, and 39 per cent were seniors in Social Studies.

Using the Army Revised Beta Test to measure pre- and post-program IQ scores, Cohen and Filipczak found that the average increase in the group of twenty-four inmates for whom they had complete data was 12.5 IQ points. They pointed out that in all except one case IQ had increased over the course of the program. These IQ gains remained when students were tested about three months later. Subtest scores were then examined to see if gains accrued disproportionately in any one area of the test for any individual, but Cohen and Filipczak concluded that in fact 'in the absence of evidence to the contrary, these IQ changes were taken to reflect across the board increases in the demonstration of ability. This applied to such areas of mental functioning as attention to detail, frustration tolerance, deductive reasoning, and acculturation' (Cohen and Filipczak, 1971, p. 132).

This was good news indeed. If provided with appropriate incentives in an educationally enriched and individualized learning environment, it was clear that even society's write-offs could make impressive academic gains. But for prison officials and government agencies, the acid test was in the follow-up data. Would the Student Educational Researchers maintain their motivation and academic performance when returned to mainstream society? Furthermore, and more importantly, would they stay out of the penal system?

In 1969, Cohen and Filipczak received more federal money, this time from the newly formed Law Enforcement Assistance Administration (LEAA), to make an evaluation of recidivism in CASE project participants. With this grant, they were able to gather information on 31 of the 41 students in the project. Twenty-six of these 31 participants were interviewed and tested to measure whether their academic gains had been maintained. Overall, they concluded that spelling, math, and reading scores were satisfactorily maintained by most students, even though they had been out of school for over two years. In terms of measuring recidivism, before analyses were undertaken, several decisions were made as to who should be included in the data set. Students who were in the program less than ninety days, and/or those who were released from CASE back into other programs or institutions before final release (rather than directly into society), were not included, reducing the sample to only 11 of the original 41 participants. Four of these 11 participants, or 36.4 per cent, recidivated within three years of their release. The group of CASE participants who served time in other penal programs before being released recidivated at the rate of 68.8 per cent. The researchers reported that according to NTS data, 76 per cent of similar juvenile delinquents recidivate during the first year. Overall, they concluded that although numbers were small, it appeared that 'the CASE program evidently delayed the delinquent's return to incarceration, but his behavior would require additional maintenance in the real world for the CASE experience to remain effective' (Cohen and Filipczak, 1971, p. 134).

Despite the fact that many CASE participants eventually ended up back in the system, Cohen and his collaborators nonetheless constructed an impassioned case for CASE. Interestingly, their argument was based not on the hard data of behavioral science – number of hours logged in programmed instruction or number of points earned in the token economy – but on their qualitative observations of the subjective improvements in the personal dignity and self-esteem of the CASE participants. As a case in point, Cohen wrote:

> When one young man came to CASE in the early part of the program, he said that there was something wrong with him. He felt that he was a misfit and could not do anything well except antisocial behaviors ... In less than one year's time, this youth learned to succeed. And when he started to succeed in academic subject matter after eight years in public school, where he had considered himself incapable and stupid, his whole approach to education and to life changed. He became a man who enjoyed the sweet smell of success. (Cohen and Filipczak, 1971, p. 141)

The termination of the CASE program coincided with the closure of the National Training School for Boys. In a letter to Cohen about a year after the program had ended, Skinner wrote that he considered the CASE project to be 'one of the most important experiments in the history of penology.'[11] The Kennedy Youth Center in Morgantown, West Virginia, replaced the NTS, and many of the principles of CASE, including the token economy, were incorporated there.[12] Cohen continued to work at the IBR and procured more grant money to spread his techniques and programs into the public school systems in Maryland and Washington, DC (see Cohen, 1972, 1976). He eventually moved to the School of Architecture and Environmental Planning at the State University of New York. Meanwhile, with the CASE programs as a model, other behavior analysts were trying their hands at behavior modification in the prison system. With grant money readily available, an arsenal of scientifically derived techniques at their disposal, and a desire to be socially relevant, they moved into cellblocks nationwide to tackle the thorny problem of how to move prisons and prisoners from incarceration to rehabilitation.

The Cellblock Token Economy

The CASE programs provided a powerful model for how to run a token economy in a total institution. The goals of CASE were educational – students earned points by meeting academic performance goals. The program did not prescribe other behavioral or institutional management agendas, although the effects of participation on general social behavior and attitudes were noted. It was perhaps the shift in emphasis away from education and skills-training and towards institutional management that ultimately created problems for behavior modification in the prison system.

    Around the same time that the CASE programs were under way, behavior analysts Carl Clements and John McKee set up the Experimental Manpower Laboratory for Corrections at the Draper Correctional Center in Elmore, Alabama. As at CASE, they were interested in education. Because their prison population consisted of adult felons, they focused on remedial academic instruction and vocational skills training. Using contingency management procedures and performance contracts, they were able to increase the quantity and quality of work performed by prisoners in the classroom. An impressive 95 per cent of the participants in their program who qualified for and took the General Educational Development test achieved their high school equivalencies, and nine participants went on to college after leaving the prison (see Clements and McKee, 1968; McKee and Clements, 1971).

    The next program at Draper was a little different. Rather than focusing on education or skills training, McKee and his behavior analytic colleague

Michael Milan made a conscious decision to 'deal with activities important for the operation of the institution' (Milan and McKee, 1976, p. 255).
They did not do so without reflection. They noted the problematic nature
of focusing on institutional management, but presented a number of jus-
tifications for doing so. They argued that correctional administrators
often see institutional management as a necessary first step before rehabilitation efforts can be undertaken. Administrators would thus be more
likely to see the practical benefits of this approach and cooperate with the
program. Also, they reasoned that inmates would not be harmed. Rather,
such a program would actually be in their best interests. Milan and McKee
pointed out that attending to directions, following instructions, accepting
constructive criticism, and working towards task completion were general
skills that would benefit inmates once they were released into the community. So what were the target behaviors at Draper? Very simply, these were
(1) getting out of bed at a determined hour; (2) making the bed; (3)
cleaning the area around the bed; and (4) maintaining a neat and well-
groomed personal appearance.

Having justified their approach, Milan and McKee then designed a
token economy program that, while focusing on different behavioral goals,
was similar in many respects to Cohen and Filipczak's CASE program. The
fifty-six participants in the token economy at Draper were housed sepa-
rately from the regular inmate population on the top floor of one of
Draper's six two-storey wings. Inmates who earned points by meeting the
behavioral goals described above could use them to gain access to a lounge,
a television room, and a poolroom. They could also use points to purchase
snack items and cigarettes at a concession stand operated for the program.
They could save up points in a program bank account and order items
from the Sears and J.C. Penney catalogues. Participants' whereabouts and
activities, as in the CASE program, were monitored by having them clock in
and out of various areas. A behavioral observation checklist was also developed and administered repeatedly throughout the 420 days of the program to investigate the effects of the token economy on the frequency of a
number of daily activities to ensure that the token economy did not result
in 'undue hardship in the form of increased deprivation of social inter-
course and/or recreational activities' (Milan and McKee, 1976, p. 269).

Milan and McKee clearly indicated that participation in the Draper
token economy was voluntary, and that even when participants overdrew
their accounts, they continued to receive all of the basic privileges
accorded to them in the regular prison environment. Clearly aware of
the controversial nature of their enterprise in their 1976 publication (by
1974 public outcry over behavior modification in prisons had reached a

high pitch), they devoted a large part of their discussion to the ethical issues involved in the implementation of rehabilitation programs in prisons, including the need for voluntary participation, community and peer review, evidence of efficacy, and public accountability. What they did not address extensively was the overall value of the rehabilitative goals, and the fact that once the token economy was discontinued, prisoners automatically reverted to baseline-level rates of behavior. Was making one's bed in exchange for a pack of cigarettes the best that could be done in the name of rehabilitation? In another program, behavior analysts were grappling with exactly this question.

The Rehabilitation Dilemma

Scott Geller was a young behavior analyst at Virginia Polytechnic Institute when, as he put it, 'there was a judge in Roanoke, maybe it was Richmond, who said everybody deserves treatment in a prison. So there is this "right to treatment" and we have these maximum security segregated inmates that are not getting treated. Would anyone like to treat them? And – I do not have a degree in clinical psychology – but that was my internship, eighteen months working with those inmates' (Geller, 2005, interview with author).

    With LEAA grant money, behavior analytic expertise, an optimistic attitude, and three colleagues (two others were operant psychologists and one was a clinical psychologist), Geller set out to design a contingency management program for the inmates of two, large, maximum security institutions – the State Penitentiary in Richmond and the Powhatan Correctional Center – starting in June of 1973. By his own account, Geller acknowledged that the rehabilitative goals of the program were limited in scope: '[T]here was no misconception that the program was designed to return offenders to society immediately as productive, law-abiding citizens' (Geller, Johnson, Hamlin, and Kennedy, 1977, p. 12). Rather, the goal was to change behaviors perceived as 'unmanageable' so that prisoners could return to the general prison population and take advantage of programs and opportunities available to them there.

    The Virginia programs were based on a contingency management approach encompassing a token economy in which inmates could earn credits exchangeable for desired goods,[13] as well as a series of stages that became less restrictive as prisoners earned their way to higher levels. To earn credits in the token economy, prisoners were expected to engage in specific education, hygiene, or job-related activities. For example, credits could be earned for keeping one's cell neat and clean, for attending to personal appearance and hygiene, and for completing components of a job assignment.

The first stage of the program included the conventional restrictions of the segregation facility, as they already existed. After moving to the second stage, prisoners gained access to programmed instruction in typing. Stage 3 participants had access to formal typing courses with an instructor, and so on. Graduation from stage 4 entitled prisoners to a transfer to a less restrictive facility and access to vocational and educational programs consistent with their individual interests and skills.

Throughout the implementation of the program, the behavior analysts encountered a number of obstacles, including the uncooperativeness of prison staff and higher-ups, high staff turnover, unhelpful prisoner attitudes towards behavior modification (which, by this time, was receiving significant negative press), as well as emerging concerns about the goals of the program. Almost any behavior that was reinforced in the token economy appeared to support compliance with prison rules, rather than rehabilitation. As political pressure mounted, one prison administrator urged Geller and his colleagues to drop all contingencies that could be construed as supporting institutionalization. Furthermore, the all-white middle-class psychologists designing the program were accused of inflicting bourgeois white values on the predominantly black prison population. As Geller put it:

> Some of the things that inmates were saying and that the ACLU was saying were, 'Well how dare you pay these guys to wear clothes! If they want to sit in their cell naked, it's their right. How dare you pay these guys to exercise – to do pushups and keep physically fit, how dare you do that? If they want to be lazy and obese, that's their right.' At this point, we said, 'What are we going to do?' ... So we said OK, what behavior could we possibly reward that couldn't be called [an example of] white middle-class values? And we came up with two classifications. One would be a verbal presentation on something the inmate would want to do that would be somewhat constructive ... we called it thinking out loud. TOL process ... The second thing was education. We would develop an educational contract with the inmates – write a poem, read a book, listen to a radio show and write a book review, anything that would improve your education ... So we thought wow! ACLU, what are you going to do about this one? (Geller, interview with author, 2005)

Thus, in response to increasing pressure to change the goals of the program, Geller and his group came up with constructive alternatives.

Despite the creativity with which the program designers met the challenge of the institutionalization versus rehabilitation dilemma, the American Civil Liberties Union (ACLU) jumped on the anti–behavior modification bandwagon.[14] Geller's program, in addition to being stymied at the more advanced levels by promises of unforthcoming transfers for stage 4 graduates, was ultimately shut down because three prisoners escaped from the program. Although prepared to go to court to defend their work, Geller and his colleagues never got the chance. In the meantime, the attention of ACLU lawyers, journalists, politicians, and the public was diverted to another, even more controversial project. The Special Treatment and Rehabilitative Training (START) program at the Federal Medical Center for Prisoners in Springfield, Missouri, soon took center stage in a national debate, not only over the use of behavior modification in the federal prison system, but over the ethical use of human subjects in behavioral research.

The Beginning and End of START

The START program was a contingency management program designed specifically for the most disruptive and aggressive prisoners in the federal correctional system. Unlike the other programs I have outlined, it was not designed or implemented directly by behavior analysts. The general overseers of the program were Norman Carlson, director of the Federal Bureau of Prisons (FBP), and Roy Gerard, assistant director and head of the Correctional Programs Division of the FBP. Gerard was a former superintendent of the National Training School for Boys and had overseen Cohen and Filipczak's CASE project. The program consultant for the START program was a PhD named Albert Scheckenback. The specific goal of the program was to work with the most violent inmates so that they could 'better control their behavior and become participants in institutional, vocational, academic, and other programs designed to help them make a successful community adjustment when released from custody' (*Behavior Modification Programs*, 1974).

START began in October of 1972 and ran for sixteen months. Out of an original pool of 99 prisoners, 19 participated in and completed the program. The program itself underwent several revisions as it unfolded, but it was basically conceptualized as a progressive stage program in which prisoners earned the right to move through stages from most restrictive to least restrictive in a typical contingency management design. Behaviors that would earn prisoners the right to move up were similar to the types of behaviors already mentioned – attending to personal hygiene, getting out of bed promptly, etc. There were, however, several aspects of the START program that were atypical. First, participation in the program was *not* voluntary. Second, the conditions at stage 1 qualified as deprivation conditions as opposed to standard prison conditions. And finally, as the program unfolded, several prisoners characterized it as 'unlawful' and 'humiliating,' and several court cases were brought forward on their behalf by lawyers from the ACLU.

As part of the pretrial procedures for a number of cases filed by prisoners in START, the court appointed a committee of expert witnesses to investigate the program. The three-person committee consisted of Harold Cohen, Nathan Azrin, and William De Risi, of the Camarillo-Neuropsychiatric Research Program in California. In responding to the court's request for their expert opinions, the committee delivered a divided assessment of START. Cohen was the most critical, stating of the program in an April 1974 article in the American Psychological Association's newsletter, *APA Monitor*: 'As a behavioral project, it is a failure. It has not produced the participation or the expected changes set forth in the original premise' (Warren, 1974, p. 3). Nathan Azrin's assessment was somewhat more equivocal. He stated in his testimony to the court that START did embody, to a substantial degree, virtually all of the major relevant principles of behavior modification as outlined by behavior analysts (Levison, 1974, p. 3). At least two of the three committee members expressed serious concern over the involuntary nature of prisoners' participation in the program. In his testimony at the oversight hearing, Norman Carlson stated that 10 of the 19 inmates who completed the program substantially benefitted from it. The program had been designed to accommodate about 30 to 35 prisoners at any given time.

Amidst considerable controversy, the program was voluntarily discontinued by the FBP on 1 March 1974, ostensibly for economic reasons. At the Oversight Hearing before the Subcommittee on Courts, Civil Liberties, and the Administration of Justice just a few days before the termination of START, Carlson remarked, 'While mistakes were undoubtedly made in developing the START program, we believe that the Bureau of Prisons profited from the experience. The effective use of programs using positive rewards for acceptable behavior can assist in developing new techniques of motivating offenders who are incarcerated' (*Behavior Modification Programs*, 1974, p. 7). Despite Carlson's assessment, the court did rule that programs such as START violated a prisoner's right to due process because the transfer of prisoners to the program was forceable and involuntary, and represented a significant change in their living conditions.

Concurrent with the termination of the START program, Senator Sam Ervin called upon the director of the LEAA, Donald Santarelli, to discontinue funding to all research programs involving behavior modification. During the course of a Senate subcommittee investigation, Ervin had determined that the agency was funding a large amount of research under the behavior modification umbrella with practically no ethical review or monitoring of the research proposals or subsequent programs. In a press release following Ervin's request, Santarelli explained that this decision had been made because 'there are no technical and professional skills on the LEAA staff to screen, evaluate, or monitor such projects' (Trotter and Warren, 1974, p. 1).

Many of these projects involved psychologists. The withdrawal of funds curtailed a considerable amount of psychological research. How did the profession of psychology and the emerging profession of behavior analysis respond?

Psychologists Respond

The day after the LEAA announcement, the American Psychological Association issued a press release. In the Association's statement, it was noted that

> behavior modification involves a large number of procedures, some of which are clearly abhorrent to psychologists as well as to the public. Other procedures, however, are humane, benign, systematic, educational, and effective. Psychologists have been in the forefront in developing and improving such procedures and applying them. The banning of these procedures will result in a regression to outmoded, unsystematic forms of inhumanity in prisons that have characterized society's past treatment of its criminal offenders.[15]

On 22 March 1974 the Board of Directors of the American Psychological Association (APA), under the presidency of Albert Bandura, recommended the formation of a task force to study the uses and misuses of behavior modification. This action was due both to 'growing public and professional concern'[16] and to pressure from APA's own Board of Social and Ethical Responsibility for Psychology (BSERP). Members of BSERP were concerned that the APA press release did not adequately represent the APA membership's views on the matter. As Fred Strassburger, psychologist and administrative officer of the Department of Social and Ethical Responsibility, later wrote to a member of the task force, 'I think

BSERP felt that some psychologists were abusing the principles of behavior modification and that APA might be too quick to come to the defense. The other side, on the other hand, were afraid that BSERP would select a panel that might be too one-sidedly critical of the "behavior modifiers." As it turned out, I don't think a better selection of panel members could have been made.'[17]

The members of what became the APA Commission on Behavior Modification included psychologists Sidney Bijou, James Holland, Leonard Krasner, Stephanie Stolz, Jerome Frank, Terence Wilson, and Serena Stier; philosopher Hugh Lacey of Swarthmore College; and two legal experts, Paul Friedman and David Wexler. Although the Commission felt that it would be desirable to have a consumer representative, their efforts to include such a representative were unsuccessful. They invited a member of the ACLU National Prison Project to attend, but were informed that the project's staff members would not have time to make a regular commitment.[18]

The Commission examined the use of behavior modification in outpatient settings, mental institutions, schools, prisons, and society in general (see Stolz and Associates, 1978; Stolz, Wienckowski, and Brown, 1975). Prisons, schools, and mental hospitals were singled out as high priority areas, and behavior analyst James Holland was appointed to consider ethical issues in prisons. In the Commission's final report, Holland authored a special chapter in which he critiqued behavioral methods as they were currently being used, arguing that 'as presently conceived, behavior modification programs in prisons, although they may ameliorate current practices, are either defective in their protection of the prisoners' rights or participate in the oppression of prisoners' (Holland, 1978, p. 86). Holland pointed out that although psychologists typically design interventions aimed at changing the individual, the more appropriate level of intervention for changing criminal behavior is societal – changing the environments in which criminal behavior occurs so that such behavior is neither necessary nor reinforcing for the individual. He noted that as used in prisons, behavior modification succeeded mainly in enforcing compliance with rules and regulations, and was not employed in the service of the individual or his future functioning in society.

Despite Holland's reservations about the use of behavior modification in prisons, and although the Commission was partly charged with considering the formulation of ethical guidelines to govern the practice of behavior modification, it decided to forego this charge. As Stephanie Stolz wrote in a memorandum to the Commission members:

I feel we should be raising key questions for people to consider, rather than laying down regulations; the questions should not prejudge legal and scientific issues, since both areas are constantly changing; the questions should apply to any sort of treatment, rather than specifically and only to behavior modification.[19]

Instead, the ultimate recommendation of the Commission was that 'persons engaged in any type of psychological intervention subscribe to and follow the ethics codes and standards of their professions,' and that the APA 'consider adopting a brief checklist of issues that could be used in the evaluation of the ethics of any psychological intervention' (Stolz and Associates, 1978, p. 114). According to the Commission, *all* psychological interventions, including but not limited to behavior modification, involve an influence and change process involving control. Techniques of behavior modification themselves 'appear to be no more or less subject to abuse and no more or less in need of ethical regulation than intervention procedures derived from any other set of principles and called by other terms' (p. 104).

Furthermore, the Commission concluded that to develop special ethical guidelines that would apply exclusively to behavior modification, thus singling it out for extra regulation, would prejudice practitioners against its use and stultify both research and applied developments within the field. Thus, in making its report to the APA, the Commission called for no special rules governing the use of behavior modification. Although the report itself was accepted by APA, it was neither endorsed nor published by the organization. This move baffled some of the Commission's own members. Hugh Lacey wrote to Stephanie Stolz inquiring 'why did the APA executive reject our report?'[20] She wrote back:

You asked about why the APA decided not to publish the Commission report. As best as I could understand it, they felt that there was no longer any interest in behavior modification, so that the report wouldn't sell very well and would lose money ... Please be clear that the APA did *accept* [italics in original] our report, as a report. That is, although APA did not want to *publish* [italics in original] the report itself, APA did accept the report and encourage us to publish it commercially. APA did not endorse our report, but I don't think any of us expected that anyway.[21]

However, despite making the case to the APA and their fellow psychologists that special regulations governing the use of behavior modification were not necessary, behavior analysts were in fact intensely concerned about the rapid and unchecked growth of their field, and its public image. In the safety of their own professional home, and on their own terms, behavior modifiers began a difficult dialogue about how to regulate themselves.

Behavior Modifiers Respond

In March of 1974, on the heels of the LEAA announcement and the formation of the APA Commission on Behavior Modification, several dozen prominent members of the rapidly expanding field of applied behavior analysis met at Drake University for an intense series of presentations and discussions. This national conference, the first of its kind, was prompted by two factors: (a) the increasing number of behavior modifiers working with more 'socially visible and controversial client populations' (Wood, 1975a, p. xv); and (b) increasing public concern about the 'growth of behavioral control methods in society' (p. xvi). Finding themselves, or others who practiced in their name, under attack for their work both in prisons and in institutions for the mentally retarded, behavior analysts recognized the need for some serious deliberations. Although this was not the first time behavior modifiers had addressed the role of behavior modification in society (see Kanfer, 1965; Krasner, 1962; Ulrich, 1967), it was, notably, the first time they came together in a professional forum.

During the course of the conference, a broad set of issues arose and were debated. These issues ranged from definitional ones (Wood, 1975b) to the possibility of national guidelines and even certification for the field and/or its practitioners (Michael, 1975; Sulzer-Azaroff, Thaw, and Thomas, 1975). Conference participants spoke on the problem of evaluating behavior analysis procedures and programs, on the need to educate the public about behavior analysis, and on questions of ethics and accountability.

What emerged from the conference was a 'set of unresolved issues' ('Professional Issues in Behavior Analysis,' 1974, p. 10). Nonetheless, the conference marked an important milestone in the group's history. In effect, behavior analysts acknowledged the need to assess their work and their role in society in a systematic and self-conscious way. In terms of numbers and impact, the field had become a force to be reckoned with. This meant that behavior analysts had to define themselves more clearly and take seriously the job of protecting the consumers of behavior modification from unqualified practitioners and ill-conceived programs, or face such regulation from outside their ranks. As one group of conference participants wrote:

> The freedom to practice behavior modification methods is clearly being threatened ... [W]e can dissociate ourselves from the whole thing by calling ourselves 'behavior analysts,' etc. But how long will it take that label to become besmirched? And who will protect the public that consumes the services of a behavior modifier? ... It is the thesis of this paper that some tool must be developed for sorting out the competent from the incompetent, or we shall all be thrown out with the bath water sullied by the malpractitioners. (Sulzer-Azaroff, Thaw, and Thomas, 1975, p. 49)

In a provocative presentation of his review of several problematic behavior modification programs in institutions for the mentally retarded, Todd Risley noted: 'This conference and other recent activity indicates that we are finally ready (indeed required) to form a profession' (Risley, 1975, p. 176). Thus, this period of public and professional scrutiny clearly set behavior analysis on the path towards professionalization. However, the issue of the protection of human subjects in behavioral research had transcended guild status and become a national concern.

Beyond Behavior Mod: The National Commission

By 1974, alarm over the treatment of human research subjects in both behavioral and biomedical research had escalated to a national concern. In 1972, the abuses of the United States Public Health Service–funded Tuskegee Study came to light in the *New York Times*. This revelation, along with awareness of a number of other similar incidents, prompted the formation of the National Commission for the Protection of Human Subjects of Biomedical and Behavioral Research in 1974. Duane Alexander, a professional staff member, recalled the role of a number of factors, including Tuskegee, in the confluence of events leading to its formation:

> Biomedical ethics had rarely received the attention from the public and from the Congress ever before that it was receiving at the time the Commission was established. This came about because of revelations of some kinds of research that had been published claiming some research had proceeded unethically – research on prisoners, research on dying patients, research on persons with mental retardation or mental disability, and then,

particularly, research on the African-American men from the Tuskegee syphilis study. (Alexander, 2004, p. 3)

Clearly, the use and misuse of behavior modification in prisons and mental hospitals was only one piece in this larger mosaic of concern, which encompassed research on a number of vulnerable populations. The Commission's mandate was to investigate issues involved in the ethical use of human subjects across a number of research areas, but the Commission paid special attention to behavioral research and behavior modification programs. They also paid special attention to the use of prisoners as research subjects (for the report on prisoners, see *National Commission*, 1976).

After a two-year examination and investigation of the nature and extent of behavioral research and behavior modification in prisons, during which Commission staff visited prisons and interviewed prisoners, they filed a report and made legislative recommendations to Congress regarding the protection of prisoners as research subjects. They recommended strictly regulating the kinds of research in which prisoners could be used as subjects, and they noted the unique conditions under which prisoners are asked to give voluntary consent. In considering the ethical issues involved, the Commission concluded that

although prisoners who participate in research affirm that they do so freely, the conditions of social and economic deprivation in which they live compromise their freedom. The Commission believes, therefore, that the appropriate expression of respect consists in protection from exploitation. Hence it calls for certain safeguards intended to reduce the elements of constraint under which prisoners give consent and suggests that certain kinds of research would not be permitted where such safeguards cannot be assured. (*National Commission*, 1976, pp. 6–7)

Specifically, the Commission recommended that research involving prisoners be restricted to the conditions particularly affecting prisoners as a class, or to studies that had the intent and reasonable probability of improving the health and well-being of the prisoners themselves. Also included in its recommendations was an outline of the basic living conditions that should be guaranteed in prisons in which research would be conducted. These conditions included, among others, adequate amounts of living space, regular access to clean and working showers, adequate recreation facilities, regular access to these facilities, and the regular issue of personal care items and clean linen.

Ultimately, the recommendations of the National Commission resulted in the stipulation that research involving prisoners as subjects must directly address or relate to the state or condition of incarceration and imprisonment, thus demonstrating some potential of benefit to the research subjects themselves, or that is must have the 'intent or reasonable probability of improving the health or well-being of the subject.'[22] The implementation and responsibilities of institutional review boards that would oversee research involving prisoners were also set out in detail in the regulations. So where did this leave behavior modification? Could behavior analysts make the case that their programs would improve the health or well-being of the subject?

Crime and Punishment

By the time the National Commission formulated its recommendations, most formal contingency management programs in prisons had been shut down or suppressed. Faced with a hostile public, nervous politicians, wary prison officials, and a withdrawal of funds, token economies as full-fledged rehabilitation schemes were stopped in their tracks. As Geller remarked retrospectively, 'We developed a leading-edge approach to motivating inmates to do better for themselves and to improve their circumstances, and even their potential beyond prison. However, the prison system was not ready, and perhaps is less ready today, to support the system we developed' (E.S. Geller, personal communication, 10 June 2003).

Concomitant with national-level attention to ethics in human subjects research, including behavioral research with prisoners, a more specific debate about the role of incarceration was unfolding. Attempts at prisoner rehabilitation on the part of behavior modifiers and others had revealed an incredibly thorny and complex set of problems that appeared to some to be insurmountable. Could voluntary participation and informed consent ever be possible in the naturally coercive prison environment? Some argued that prisoners gave up their right to 'choose' treatment when they committed their offence. Others argued that the right to treatment had put the right to refuse treatment in jeopardy. In the deliberations of the APA Commission on Behavior Modification, legal expert David Wexler noted that the prison has at least four goals: detention, deterrence, retribution, and rehabilitation. Further, he pointed out that 'the older legal view that society had a compelling state interest to change behavior, hence to provide treatment, is giving way to a newer emerging approach. This approach takes the position that criminal behavior should result in appropriate retribution for a limited period of time.'[23]

Supporters of this new, emerging approach cited evidence that rehabilitation had failed to live up to its promise, and that data from prison treatment programs consistently showed no difference in subsequent crime rates between inmates given treatment and those who sat idly in their cells. Coupled with concerns that some of the methods used under the guise of treatment were in fact inhumane or supported the goals of the jailer rather than the jailed, the pendulum of public sentiment shifted from a treatment model back to a justice model of incarceration.[24] The cultural opening that had provided an 'in' for behavior modifiers and others to ply their trade in the name of rehabilitation, gradually closed. In 1977, Senator Edward Kennedy proposed a bill to restructure criminal sentencing in which the purpose of imprisonment was limited to providing 'just punishment for the offence.' Notably, the language of treatment and rehabilitation was completely absent. In reviewing this turn of events, psychologist John Monahan, a fellow in psychology and law at Harvard University, wrote:

> There is little doubt that the pendulum is on the move and that prisons will once again be a place where people go to be punished rather than cured. Enforced rehabilitation and indeterminate sentences were noble social experiments. But, like prohibition, their time has come and gone. (Monahan, 1977, p. 13)

Thus, in retrospect, those behavior modifiers who did venture beyond the box to the prison cellblock experienced only a brief window of opportunity. The tide of public sentiment that advanced their work in the late 1960s just as quickly curtailed it in the mid-1970s. After the thousands of dollars spent trying to treat inmates and reform prisons, it seemed retribution had trumped rehabilitation. Although some argued that rehabilitation as a social experiment had failed, behavior modifiers argued that they had not been given sufficient opportunity, under adequate conditions, to prove the worth of their techniques. Behavior modifiers experienced, sometimes acutely, the powerful influence of their social context. As society's values shifted, attitudes towards their work changed. Instead of providing a solution, behavior modification became part of the problem.

In the end, behavior modifiers gained some valuable experience from their participation in the prison business. As they exchanged the role of scientist for that of technologist of behavior, they found they could not hide behind the veil of value-neutrality. As Scott Wood, the host of the Drake Conference, astutely remarked, 'We now are confronted by a public, by governing agencies, and by other colleagues whose concern is not whether our methods and principles are scientifically valid, but rather what we intend to do with them. It is our values, not our science, that are being questioned' (Wood, 1975b, p. 27). Whereas CASE had been on relatively safe ground using behavior modification to foster academic achievement and education, as behavior analysts succumbed to the practical and political exigencies of the prison milieu, they increasingly designed programs to create more tractable prisoners.

Behavior analysts were thrust into a maelstrom of conflicting value systems. Were they servants of the state, or the patient? The prison official or the inmate? Were they using a technology of behavior to straightjacket the problem patient or emancipate the patient's potential? Further, how could they safeguard their techniques so that practitioners with questionable aims could be regulated? How could they give behavior modification away without losing control over their work? As James Holland wrote of this dilemma:

> [B]ehavior modification techniques are cumulative. After the technique is developed, the scientist can move on to dealing with new problems; the procedures, once developed, no longer require professional personnel ... Therefore, responsibility for its use does not rest solely with a small identifiable professional group guided by an ethical code and easily held accountable by society. (Holland, 1976, p. 72)

In fact, one eventual outcome of this period of public scrutiny was the genesis of a certification movement among behavior analysts. The co-optation and implementation of behavioral technologies by those outside their ranks forced behavior analysts to begin the process of forming an 'identifiable professional group' that would monitor and regulate its practitioners.

Before this, however, the process of spreading behavior modification would continue. As Holland noted, behavioral procedures, once developed and tested, no longer required professional oversight or professional personnel. The purview of the technology of behavior was about to expand even further, and in doing so would subtly change the very nature of self-understanding in American society. North Americans were about to learn how to be their own behavior analysts.

chapter 5

How to *Really* Win Friends and Influence People: Skinnerian Principles in Self-Help

The solution to many neurotic problems often consists of doing something to bring behavior to an end instead of simply ending it. Is this the difference between self-management by exercising the 'will' (just stopping a bad habit) and by changing the environmental contingencies?

Skinner, 1980, p. 96

Does self-reinforcement really work? Even the reader who has completed a successful project may ask this question: was it the self-reinforcement or was it the will-power that made the difference?

Watson and Tharp, 1972, p. 241

Skinner became famous – and notorious – for using his behavioral principles on himself. As he noted, 'I have, I think, made good use of my analysis of behavior in managing my own life ... Can the psychoanalysts and the cognitive and humanistic psychologists say as much?' (Skinner, 1980, p. 75). Skinner took particular advantage of his approach in the design of the basement study of his modest home on Old Dee Road, a few miles from Harvard Square. In this subterranean retreat, where he did most of his writing, he constructed a variety of gadgets and devices that allowed him to control his environment, and thus his behavior. For example, for many years Skinner rose early to write, often going directly from his bed to his desk. He would then switch on his desk lamp, which was connected to a timer. When his writing time was up, the timer would switch off his desk lamp, signaling the end of the writing period. In effect, the light was a discriminative stimulus for writing behavior. For Skinner, setting up environmental contingencies for personal self-management was a natural outcome of behavior analysis.[1]

As Skinner's system expanded into a full-fledged technology of behavior and behavior modifiers used their expertise to change the behavior of others in institutional settings, they also explored the potential of their techniques in everyday life. If time out could be used on the psychiatric ward, why not in the home? Why not use stimulus control in a personal weight-loss program? How about a self-designed and implemented token economy? Could people be taught to be their own behavior analysts?

As many writers, both scholarly and popular, have pointed out, the practice and principles of behavior modification have existed throughout time and place: 'Commonsense notions of the ways in which reward and punishment can change behavior have existed since time immemorial' (Stolz, Wienckowski, and Brown, 1975, p. 1027). Money is the most obvious generalized reinforcer around, and tokens or credits are little more than money substitutes. The power of positive reinforcement has been experienced by anyone who has ever become hooked on lottery tickets after a small win, or rewarded themselves with a vacation after completing a difficult assignment. Given that the principles used by behavior analysts in their work 'are available to and in fact are universally used by virtually all people at all times' (Stuart and Davis, 1972, p. 75), how did applied behavior analysts lay claim to a body of specialized knowledge and a set of specialized techniques, and then export them to the public? How did they negotiate the tricky balance of 'giving behavior analysis away'[2] while maintaining their professional authority in the process?

In part, behavior analysts negotiated this balance by using the cultural authority and practical tools of science, and by capitalizing on the voracious American appetite for self-help recipes formulated by scientific experts.[3] Systematic observation, measurement, control, and precise monitoring of behavior took the behavior analytic system beyond common sense and placed it in the hands of behavior experts. As behavior analysts themselves wrote: 'The principles of behavior modification *codify* and *organize* common sense, showing under what conditions and in what circumstances each aspect of "common sense" should be applied' (Stolz et al., 1975, p. 1029, italics added). The techniques of behavior modification, although in many cases topographically similar to everyday practices, were scientifically derived and tested – based on findings from the experimental analysis of behavior, which itself was conducted in what sociologist Thomas Gieryn would call a 'truth spot' – the scientist's laboratory.[4] The application of these principles to dieting, parenting, and assertiveness training thus benefitted from their place of provenance. The fact that the principles were systematically tested in the laboratory of the psychological scientist afforded them significant cultural currency.

Behavior analysts also distinguished their techniques from common sense by formulating a specific language that set their advice apart and marked it as scientific, or at least technical. This was the language of positive and negative reinforcement, stimulus generalization, stimulus control, aversive consequences, functional relationships, and self-control. In using this language, they also faced the problem of reverse translation. Having translated common sense into technical language, they then had to translate it back in order to appeal to their consumers. For example, in *Behavior Modification: The Scientific Way to Self-Control*, author William Budd wrote:

> Psychologists frequently talk about 'stimulus control' of a certain behavior. By this they mean that the particular behavior is usually associated with such events as the end of a meal, with driving, with watching television, with visiting friends, and with other specific situations. (Budd, 1973, p. 61)

Sometimes their audiences appropriated the technical language as a way of rebelling against the techniques. Israel Goldiamond, in writing of his attempts to help a student in one of his classes develop better study habits, reported her reaction to his attempts: 'I know what you're up to. You want that desk to assume stimulus control over me. I'm not going to let any piece of wood run my life for me' (Goldiamond, 1965, p. 854).

With the use of the concept of self-control, behavior analysts signified not only a change in language, but a change in approach. Willpower, insight, and actualization were out, behavioral self-control was in. Shedding a few pounds or giving up cigarettes was no longer a matter of exercising willpower, gaining insight into unconscious motivations, or achieving self-actualization. Behavior analysts highlighted the limitations of these inner-focused approaches: 'Many of the humanistically oriented techniques ... fail to provide self-controlling skills. Too often the focus is excessively insightful rather than "outsightful." That is, the person focuses on historical understandings and current interpretations rather than on the functional relationships between his own behavior and the immediate environment' (Thoresen and Mahoney, 1974, p. 140). Building self-control became a matter of analyzing and arranging one's environment in specific ways to maximize the probability of the desired behavior change.

Behavior analysts applied the techniques of self-control to a wide range of personal problems in the 1970s. These included overeating, lack of assertiveness, fears and phobias, poor study habits, marital and sexual problems, smoking, and parenting. But the impulse to train people to be their own behavior analysts had started earlier. As Israel Goldiamond wrote to Skinner in 1962: 'If operant procedures are to be used [outside the laboratory], then they should be used frankly, and in on-going analysis, to shape self-control. So, I have been counseling a) obese students, b) students who are flunking out of school, and c) marital problems.'[5]

Undoubtedly, others had also been using the principles of behavior analysis to help others help themselves with a variety of life's problems. In fact, by 1976, there were so many self-help programs based on behavior modification that one behavior therapist suggested that professional regulations be developed to help monitor the quality and effectiveness of self-administered 'non-prescription' behavior therapies. In 1976, psychologist Gerald Rosen noted the proliferation of the 'self-help' behavior modification literature and called for increased quality control, worrying that the spirit of empirical rigor so central to the field was being diluted as behavior modifiers jostled for their piece of the self-help pie (Rosen, 1976).

Although Rosen's recommendations for monitoring this literature were not adopted, his article and the rejoinder to it written by Israel Goldiamond highlighted the genre's rise to prominence. As behavior modifiers began to see the success of their efforts in closed environments such as psychiatric wards and classrooms, a desire to promote the use of their principles in everyday life quickly ensued. As Harold Cohen told journalist and author of *Behavior Mod*, Philip Hilts, in a *Washington Post* article in 1973: 'Unlike sex, you can do it yourself and it's exciting. You can turn yourself on' (Hilts, 1973b, p. 21). In 1973, behavior analyst William Budd wrote, 'Anyone can become a more proficient behavioral engineer for his own behavior' (p. 94).

Among the range of behaviors available to the behavioral engineer, overeating (not sex) was one of the earliest problems to be tackled. According to the behavior modifiers, the key to a slimmer you lay not in the power of your will, but in your ability to arrange environmental contingencies. Skinner once again reached popular audiences, in yet another incarnation: diet guru. A tongue-in-cheek article entitled 'Thinner with Skinner' appeared in *Cosmopolitan* magazine in 1978, chronicling the author's radical weight-loss method that, although it drew little on Skinnerian techniques, nonetheless ended with the plea, 'Help, Professor Skinner, help me' (Sokolov, 1978, p. 192). Unbeknownst to readers of *Cosmopolitan*, Skinnerians had been helping overeaters since at least the mid-1960s.

Self-Control and the Human Eater

In 1965 an excited testimonial arrived on Charles Ferster's desk at the Institute for Behavioral Research in Silver Spring, Maryland:

> Dear Dr. Ferster,
> I am a psychiatric nurse in charge of Unit 9 at Patton State Hospital ... Since November of 1964 we have made practical use of operant conditioning procedures in an open unit ... In this experiment in operant conditioning, we of nursing service attempt to shape and control the behavior of chronic schizophrenic patients. When I was in the program a little over two months, I decided that if I expected the patients to change old habits, I had better start on myself ... I weighed 263 pounds and was sorely in need of changing my eating habits. It occurred to me that operational [*sic*] procedures could apply in my case. I developed self-control in eating much the same as you have recorded in your paper 'The control of eating.' I have demonstrated that this method does work![6]

How well did the method work? Nurse Norma Fullgrabe lost ninety-five pounds using Ferster's method. Was 'The control of eating' a miracle diet? Had a behavior analyst discovered the cure for obesity?

In 1962, Ferster and two of his colleagues at the Indiana University Medical Center published an article in which they provided an analysis of eating behavior and outlined strategies to control this behavior. In their words, 'This report is an account of the application of some elementary general principles of reinforcement theory to the analysis of the behavior of the human eater' (Ferster, Nurnberger, and Levitt, 1962/1977, p. 309). Their report was actually based on an experimental diet control program that Ferster carried out with a number of 'human eaters' – twelve nurses at the Medical Center, ranging in age from twenty-four to sixty-five years, who had presumably self-identified as wanting help with dieting and weight loss.[7]

So what did the nurses do to lose weight, or as Ferster and Fullgrabe put it, to develop self-control in eating? The researchers outlined four steps: (1) determining what variables influence eating; (2) determining how these variables can be manipulated; (3) identifying the unwanted effects – or ultimate aversive consequences (UACs) of overeating; and (4) arranging a method of developing required self-control – perhaps the most challenging task, at times requiring so 'drastic a change in behavior' that reinforcing by successive approximations became necessary (Ferster, Nurnberger, and Levitt, 1962/1977, p. 310). Of note was Ferster's insistence that the program was not about developing willpower or some other internal property. Developing self-control, like any other behavioral problem, was a matter of arranging the environment and manipulating conditions to make some behaviors unlikely (eating) and others more likely (not eating).

Ferster asked the nurses to do a number of things in the first four weeks of the program. First, they were asked to talk about and write down all of the negative consequences of overeating, to develop a 'fluent verbal repertoire about the relevant aversive consequences' (Ferster, Nurnberger, and Levitt, 1962/77, p. 311). This involved group discussions and writing assignments in which the nurses disclosed feelings of social rejection, personal sensitivity about being overweight, hurt over sarcastic comments, frustration with dieting preoccupation, and other aversive events and emotions. Ferster emphasized the importance of this step of the program, especially in terms of bringing the UACs of overeating into more direct contact with overeating itself. Nurses were instructed to verbalize or imagine these consequences in situations where the temptation to overeat was high. Conversely, when self-control was exercised, these UACs diminished in a process of negative reinforcement. Ferster wrote: 'In the case of our subjects, the development of the UAC was one of the major parts of the practical program.'[8]

The nurses also kept daily logs of everything they ate along with calculations of caloric, fat, carbohydrate, and protein intake. During this phase of the program, they followed a maintenance diet so that they could solidify their self-control strategies before actually attempting to lose weight. Controlling the rate of weight loss was deemed essential to ensure that self-control procedures would not be overwhelmed by the temptation to eat when severely deprived of calories. Practically speaking, this meant that the researchers specified a weight loss of no more than one pound a week 'even though all of them [the nurses] were willing to cut their diets more stringently in order to achieve a greater rate of weight loss.'[9] Nurses were also instructed in the principle of stimulus control, in which they were taught to gradually restrict the range of situations, places, and times in which they ate. The idea of prepotent repertoires was introduced – engaging in a competing activity like going for a walk or to a movie when the disposition to eat was high. Taking advantage of satiation effects was also recommended: housewives who nibbled while preparing the evening meal were instructed to shift meal preparation to the period of time immediately following lunch (evidently, the idea of asking their husbands to make dinner was ahead of its time!).

Despite Ferster's interest in the project and its apparent success (at least in the case of Norma Fullgrabe), this early treatise on the control of eating was relegated to an extremely obscure publication outlet, the *Journal of Mathetics*, and received little attention. The journal was the brainchild of Thomas Gilbert, who worked briefly with Skinner on educational issues in the late 1950s. Gilbert coined the term 'mathetics' to refer to the systematic application of reinforcement theory to the analysis of complex behavior repertoires, but published only two self-financed issues of the journal before it folded (see Kazdin, 1978, pp. 244–5). Furthermore, it appears that Ferster left the problems of the human eater behind when he moved from Indiana to Maryland. The idea of applying behavioral strategies to the problem of overeating, however, soon caught on.[10]

Slim Chance

One of the most widely referenced and well-known weight-control manuals of the 1970s was Richard Stuart and Barbara Davis's *Slim Chance in a Fat World: Behavioral Control of Obesity* (1972). Stuart, a behavioral psychologist in the School of Social Work at the University of Michigan, influenced by Ferster's 1962 article, designed his own behavioral treatment program involving eight patients and reported the results in a 1967 publication (Stuart, 1967). In this article he wrote, 'The behavioral processes involved in a person's control of himself are the same as those one would use in controlling the behavior of others' (p. 357). Self-control, in Stuart's view, involved controlling one's own behavior in the same way one might control the behavior of anyone else. A self-administered behavioral program to treat overeating was clearly possible.

In their 1972 manual, Stuart and Davis made their self-help philosophy clear from the outset: 'the environment rather than the man is the agent of control of human behavior' (Stuart and Davis, 1972, p. 62). They explained that their approach was based on the principles of behavior modification, and introduced their technical language immediately. They described in detail four classes of antecedent conditions and four classes of consequences that would affect the probability of overeating. Thus, the reader learned of discriminative, facilitative, instructional, and potentiating stimuli, as well as positive and negative reinforcers, punishment, and extinction. The reader was then taken through a rather elaborate series of steps employing these principles in the behavioral control of overeating.

The reader first learned to narrow the span of situational cues associated with eating. That is, readers were told to arrange to eat only in one place in one room and not to engage in any other activities while eating, such as reading or watching television. The second step was 'constructing an environment free of stimuli that might cause overeating' (p. 79), or, more simply stated, putting temptation out of reach. If possible, the dieter should remove tempting food from the house and increase the 'response cost of eating' (p. 81) by setting up procedures which would make it difficult to eat high-calorie foods intended for other family members.

Another important component of the *Slim Chance* program was the use of self-administered positive reinforcement following the completion of eating and exercise requirements or weight loss. In fact, the authors recommended a self-administered token economy approach. Dieters were encouraged to set up a token reinforcement menu in which behavioral goals such as following the diet for one meal (or three meals, or one week) would earn tokens which could then be exchanged for tangible, presumably non-consumable, rewards. In their sample menu, they suggested an award of 3 tokens for following one's diet for one meal, or 100 tokens for following one's diet for seven consecutive days. The successful dieter could then exchange 500 tokens for a new dress. Twenty-five tokens might buy an extra babysitter for three hours during the day (Stuart and Davis, p. 94). The power of social reinforcement was also highlighted; the weight-reducer was advised to enlist the help of others, and to discuss her efforts only with those sympathetic to her goals. Finally, the authors provided some more advice from their clinical experience, noting, 'It is wise ... *not to undertake a weight control program shortly before a holiday*' (italics in original), as there may be 'concentrated social pressure to eat excessively' (p. 96). With this sage advice and your new, lighter step, you might also be ready to undertake further improvement – how about becoming more assertive?

Behaving Assertively

In 1970, Robert Alberti and Michael Emmons published their popular book *Your Perfect Right: A Guide to Assertive Behavior.* Between 1970 and 1978, *Your Perfect Right* underwent thirteen printings and two editions.[11] Becoming more assertive became a simple matter of practicing new, assertive, behavior patterns.

Interestingly, Alberti and Emmons, rather than presenting themselves explicitly as behavior modifiers, couched their program in the language of self-actualization and personal growth. Often, however, this language received concrete behavioral translation. In fact, in their discussion of goal-setting, Alberti presented 'A Behavioral Model for Personal Growth' based on Carl Rogers's three components of a healthy personality: openness to experience, existential living, and trust in the organism. Alberti accomplished this humanist-cum-behaviorist sleight of hand by providing explicit behavioral operationalizations of Rogers's concepts. To become increasingly open to experience, for example, one might set as a behavioral goal studying a new language or culture, watching a bird soar on the wind's current, or tasting a new food. This was an interesting strategy for capitalizing on the popularity of humanistic psychology in this period without straying too far from the book's behaviorist underpinnings.

Despite this humanistic gloss, Alberti and Emmons acknowledged that through their experience with 'hundreds of clients' in assertiveness training, and 'countless reports' from colleagues and readers, what was needed to become more assertive was not a change in attitude, or a will to change. They wrote, 'We won't ask you to wake up some morning and say, "Today I am a new, assertive person!" The key to developing assertiveness is *practice of new behavior patterns*' (Alberti and Emmons, 1974, p. 58, italics in original).

To practice these new behavior patterns, readers were presented with fifteen steps (seventeen by the 1990 edition!). They were instructed to observe their own behavior, to keep track of assertive behaviors in a log or diary, to set small, low-risk behavioral goals, to imagine appropriate assertive responses, to rehearse these responses imaginally, and then to try them out in role play. The authors specified that these last three steps should be repeated as often as necessary to 'shape behavior' to a point where the new response could be tried out in vivo. After trying out the new behaviors, the final step was to institute a reliable program of self-reinforcement in order to maintain the newly developed assertive behavior. Self-actualization had little to do with this concrete approach. Rather, feeling self-actualized was a by-product or consequence (perhaps even a reinforcer!) of these new behavior patterns.

Be Your Own Behavior Modifier

Behavior analysts did not limit their advice to specific problems such as overeating or lack of assertiveness. Part of the beauty of behavior mod lay in its complete transparency and the ease with which it could be applied to any behavior-change project – it was a completely transferable technology, with almost infinite applications. In 1978, behavior analysts Gary Martin and Joseph Pear wrote a general how-to book entitled *Behavior Modification: What It Is and How to Do It.* The book proved incredibly popular, generating seven editions.

Martin and Pear devoted a chapter to self-control procedures and pointedly reminded the reader that 'behavior, as this book has constantly emphasized, is controlled by the environment – not by inner forces such as "will-power." So your bad habits exist not because you lack will power, but because they are supported by "bad" contingencies of reinforcement in your environment … What others might call will power is referred to by behavior modifiers as techniques of *self-control*' (Martin and Pear, 1978, p. 366, italics in original). They aptly noted that in the case of self-control, the individual assumed the major responsibility for carrying out the program – that is, arranging his/her own contingencies. They avowed as how this might lead to a difficulty called 'short-circuiting of contingencies.' Short-circuiting referred to the self-administration of reinforcers in the *absence* of the desired behavior change. But to reiterate, the solution to short-circuiting was not to lay blame or to self-admonish. The solution was to set up such powerful environmental contingencies that short-circuiting would be less and less likely to occur. One had to write willpower out of the equation; obliterate agency with determinism in the service of self-control.

Assuming that you could avoid the dangers of short-circuiting, Martin and Pear then guided readers through a self-modification protocol. The first step was to identify a problem and its controlling variables. What contingencies reinforced the problem behavior? The next step involved 'baselining' the problem – that is, monitoring and recording when, where, and how often the problem behavior occurred. Martin and Pear suggested that if you found yourself less-than-motivated to record your own behavior, you could arrange for your friends to reinforce your recording behavior with encouragement. The reader was then instructed on how to draw up a behavioral contract that would specify the problem and goal in behavioral terms, the reinforcers to be used and how they would be delivered, and any potential problems and their resolutions. The authors concluded optimistically with: 'In short, many people can be their own behavior therapist' (p. 382).

Watson and Tharp, in their 1972 volume *Self-Directed Behavior: Self-Modification for Personal Adjustment,* took a similar tack to Martin and Pear in dealing with the thorny problem of willpower. They encouraged readers to see the will, not as something separate from self-control (or self-reinforcement, as they put it), but as functionally equivalent to it. They wrote:

> Scientific principles of behavior can be used to increase your range of self-determination. Self-determination can be strengthened by managing the environmental conditions that affect it. Therefore, willpower *is not something separate* [italics in original] that must be invoked to explain self-modification. It *is* [italics in original] self-modification. Learning to increase self-determined behavior is learning will. (Watson and Tharp, 1972, p. 249)

To Thine Own Self Be True?

One of the curious features of the Skinnerian self-help literature was the persistence of the notion of self. Despite translating willpower into self-control and emphasizing environment over attitude, the necessity of a self to figure out and set up the appropriate environmental contingencies remained. If, as Skinner suggested, we can neither blame the self for its mistakes, nor accept praise for deeds well done, how do the very specific contingencies responsible for self-control get set up in the first place? If the self is not agentic, where does this all start? Goldiamond's description of how to change one's own behavior demonstrates this conundrum: 'If you want a specified behavior from yourself, set up the conditions which you know will control it ... Within this context, the Greek maxim, "Know thyself," translates into "Know thy behaviors, know thy environment, and know the functional relation between the two"' (Goldiamond, 1973, p. 270). Remaining salient is the knower, the self, who can perform the functional analysis and execute strategies based on the results.

In his book *Science and Human Behavior,* Skinner asked, 'What is meant by the "self" in self-control or self-knowledge? When a man jams his hands into his pockets to keep himself from biting his nails, *who* is controlling *whom?*' (Skinner, 1953, p. 283, italics in original). He ultimately defined self as 'a functionally unified set of responses' and argued that the ultimate source of self-control was not the self, but the society in which this 'unified set of responses' resided. Skinner remarked, 'It is easy to tell an alcoholic that he can keep himself from drinking by throwing away available supplies of alcohol; the principal problem is to get him to do it' (Skinner, 1953, p. 240). He explained that when society sets up sanctions against alcoholism (or any other sets of behaviors), it provides automatic reinforcement of behavior which controls drinking because such behavior reduces conditioned aversive stimulation (i.e., throwing away alcohol reduces the social disapproval incurred by keeping it and drinking it). Skinner thus concluded, 'It appears, therefore, that society is responsible for the larger part of the behavior of self control' and 'little ultimate control remains within the individual' (p. 240). His conclusions revealed the radical nature of his underlying philosophy, which was truly, ontologically, agency-less.

I would argue that in large part, the self-control literature spawned by Skinner's system was not based on Skinner's own radical philosophy, but relied instead on the practical value of Skinner's techniques. To be one's own behavior analyst, one did not need to be a *radical* behaviorist, nor in fact was the idea even introduced. In fact, in order to sell behaviorism as self-help, many used the opposite strategy. Alberti and Emmons co-opted Carl Rogers, providing a behavioral spin on openness to experience and existential living. Thoresen and Mahoney referred to the techniques of behavioral self-control as both 'empirical humanism' and 'applied humanism' (Mahoney and Thoresen, 1974; Thoresen and Mahoney, 1974). They explained that the person who knows and manages the many environments that influence him or her is demonstrating personal dignity, and armed their readers with the tellingly anti-Skinnerian mantra 'Power to the person' (Mahoney and Thoresen, 1974). This was likely based on their personal rejection of radical behaviorist philosophy and a reaction against Skinner's polemic in *Beyond Freedom and Dignity*, which had recently attracted the public's attention.

The Science of Self-Help

In the 1960s and particularly in the 1970s, behavior analysts exported their techniques of measurement, observation, and functional analysis from the laboratory, clinic, and classroom to an eager public. They did so by parlaying their science into self-help and using their technical language to dress up common sense in scientific garb, simultaneously capitalizing on the appeal of common sense and the cultural authority of science to make the medicine go down. In this period, everybody could learn to be their own behavior modifier. The key was to tap into the power of environmental contingencies; to help oneself, one had to change one's environment.

Behavior modification was particularly well suited to the self-help genre. A unique aspect of this new therapy was that unlike other forms, such as psychoanalysis or Rogerian client-centered therapy, the individual could in fact be his or her own behavior modifier – no therapist required. Since the key to behavior change was changing one's environment in specifiable ways, the individual could learn a few simple principles, apply them systematically to his or her own situation, and behavior change should ensue. However, the behavior modifiers subtly changed or revised existing understandings of self-help. First, self-help became transformed almost seamlessly into self-control. To help oneself one had to develop self-control. No longer was self-control a matter of exerting willpower, resolve, self-restraint, or impulse control. It became, in behavior analytic language, the person's own manipulation of the environmental contingencies required to produce desired behavior change. Or, as Thoresen and Mahoney put it in their 1974 book *Behavioral Self-Control*: 'A person displays self-control when in the relative absence of immediate external constraints, he engages in behavior whose previous probability has been less than that of alternatively available behaviors' (p. 12).

I would further argue that the refinement and use of the language of control by specialists in behavior modification actually influenced both the collective and individual definition of self-help. The emergence of a specific self-help language couched in technical, behavioral terms, changed the way behavior modification was socially and politically negotiated, and culturally evaluated. In creating this language, behavior modifiers produced a powerful new means through which the public could talk about, discuss, debate, and challenge practices that had, in fact, existed in non-codified form for some time. In turn, this public discourse affected the very practices and practitioners themselves, solidifying a label and an identity that, before this time, had been less distinct and whose boundaries had been less well defined.

In suggesting that behavior modifiers in this period developed and used a new language of behavioral control that codified and objectified common-sense practices, I am not suggesting that this was, in fact, the sum total of their innovation. Behavior modifiers went beyond common sense by using science to evaluate, systematize, and codify existing practices, thus making them more efficient, effective, and scientific. As behavioral psychologist Alan Kazdin put it, 'Observing one's own behavior is a common event. Few persons, however, observe their own behavior in an organized, systematic fashion' (Kazdin, 1974, p. 218). And as Harold Cohen expressed it in the *Washington Post*, 'Basically, there is nothing new in all of this … they are just Grandma's rules … There are laws of behavior as there are laws of gravity. We are just trying to use them systematically' (as cited in Hilts, 1973b, p. 41).

Thus, in selling their science to the public, behavior modifiers were able to leverage the cultural authority of science, the power of the laboratory as truth spot, and the accepted scientific tropes of careful observation, measurement, and control to their advantage, without abandoning the appeal to common sense. I would suggest further that it was the behavior modifiers' codifying of common sense in the behavioral language of control that was essential in producing and solidifying their own professional identities.

Thus, applied behavior analysis entered popular discourse in the 1970s as behavior modification, and linguistically codified practices that, although previously and universally applied, had never been talked about in this precise way. Armed with a vocabulary and the principles it described, behavior modifiers were able to specify a new form of self-help – self-control. Additionally, the new language offered a redefinition/ translation of several familiar terms. Self-control became an exercise in contingency management, not willpower. Self-awareness became self-observation, as in recording the frequency of a behavior and its controlling variables. In addition to the obvious social, and to some extent moral, implications of these changes, the language itself facilitated a conversation that could not have existed without this vocabulary.

To borrow from Kurt Danziger's discussion of behavioral psychology in his book *Naming the Mind* (1997), 'behavior modifier' was now given the distinction of designating a certain kind of professional. It supplied an identity label that challenged others to either accept or reject this class of behavioral engineers and their work. Whether feared, hated, or embraced, behavior modification could be talked about in a way that it hadn't been talked about before. No longer a moving target, it became an identifiable and distinct set of practices susceptible to both condemnation and praise.

But did the language of behavior modification change the experience of self-control, or social control for that matter, in any psychologically meaningful way? Did this change in psychological language signify psychological change in its own right, as Graham Richards has suggested (Richards, 1996)? In his popular 1974 book *Behavior Mod*, journalist Philip Hilts predicted that this would be the case:

> The mod squadders keep graphs on themselves, their children, their friends. They analyze politics, government, and laws by behavioral principles. The world is a different place, with a different set of boundaries, structures, and meanings for the mod squadders ... For a society obsessed with efficient tools, with getting results, the neat systems of the behaviorists will be hard to resist. (Hilts, 1974, p. 17)

With almost thirty years of historical hindsight, it is clear that Hilts's mod squadders have not single-handedly changed the world. Practically speaking, most of us do not keep graphs of our own behavior, or self-administer tokens for a pound lost.[12] These practices may well be prescribed by a behaviorally oriented practitioner, or used in institutional settings. Worth considering, however, are the ways in which changes in linguistic practices affect both the activities of psychologists and their social impact. Without its own language, applied behavior analysis may not have maintained an identity separate from the rest of behavioral psychology. Without this identity, the field's social impact would have been hard to discern. The process of cultural evaluation that ensued was in large part dependent on the availability of a professional target with its own set of specialized terms. These terms differentiated behavior modification from common sense and from other forms of self-help. Whether this language helped or hindered the behavior analytic enterprise is a matter of ongoing debate.

In 1969, APA president and cognitive psychologist George A. Miller asked his colleagues to consider more thoughtfully and thoroughly how psychological science could be used as a means of promoting human welfare (Miller, 1969). He argued that the most effective way for scientific psychology to influence public psychology was not to devise technologies that could be placed into the hands of 'powerful men' [sic], but to devise 'a new and different public conception of what is humanly possible and what is humanly desirable,' which would 'entail a change in our conception of ourselves and of how we live and love and work together' (p. 1066). He then went on to roundly criticize the psychology of behavior control, not for its lack of scientific validity, but for its corrosive effect on the public perception of psychology. 'In the public view, I suspect, all this talk of controlling behavior comes across as unpleasant, if not actually threatening ... the simple fact that many psychologists keep talking about control is having an effect on public psychology' (p. 1068). He then warned of the unfortunate consequences that could befall society if the science of control were to fall into the hands of an industrial or bureaucratic elite.

As I have already shown, Miller was not alone in his concerns about behavior control in this period. It is clear that by the 1970s even the technologists of behavior knew that they had to soften their language to make inroads into public psychology, and that they could not force their technology unilaterally on unwilling subjects. As Rebecca Lemov has written in her account of social scientists as human engineers in the first half of the twentieth century, '[T]he work of human engineers shows that the only method that will bring about a *true* change of being, a moment at which there is a shift, would be a cooperative one' (Lemov, 2005, p. 248). By appropriating the self-help genre, subtly eliding self-help with self-control, and then adding a humanistic gloss, the be-your-own behavior modifiers were able to enlist the cooperation of their consumers. They also enacted a small but significant shift in their message: despite radical behaviorism's insistence to the contrary, the *self* control of behavior control *was* possible.

chapter 6

Living the Dream:
Walden Two and the Laboratory of Life

Communal orders represent major social experiments in which new or radical theories of human behavior, motivation, and interpersonal relations are put to the test. Social science has rarely had 'laboratories' of the scale and scope of utopian communities.

Kanter, 1972, p. viii

In 1948, B.F. Skinner published a utopian novel called *Walden Two*. Despite his early aspirations to become a novelist, this short book was the only work of fiction he ever published. In it he described a pastoral community in which both interpersonal and human–environment relationships were engineered with the use of behavioral principles, a community where the workday could be shortened to four hours with no loss in productivity, where leisure could be spent in a variety of rewarding ways, and where no one would want for anything or feel coerced into performing undesirable tasks. Why was Skinner seized with a surge of utopianism so early in his career? In a letter written to an interested inquirer eleven years later, he remarked:

> I came to write *Walden Two* in the following way. In the spring of 1945 I sat next to a woman at a dinner party who had a son and son-in-law in the South Pacific. I remarked casually, 'What a shame that these young men, with such crusading spirits, must come back and sign up in a society in which they do not really believe.' She asked me what I would have them do instead ... She insisted that I write these ideas up for the benefit of young people ... I insisted that I had other deadlines to meet, but she was quite adamant. I did meet one such deadline on June 1, and then to my surprise

began to write *Walden Two* which I finished within seven weeks. The only preparation for writing it had been a sporadic interest in community experiments in the United States, and extensive reading of Thoreau.[1]

Skinner had no idea, upon writing *Walden Two,* that it would sell as well as it eventually did or that it would inspire would-be communitarians in the 1960s to originate Walden Two–type communities (see Kinkade, 1973, 1994). In fact, he had a hard time getting it published, it did not sell well when it first appeared, and he remarked that he didn't pay much attention to it himself or use it in his courses until many years later (Elms, 1981, p. 476). The reformist and utopian impulses he expressed in *Walden Two* required the emergence of the counterculture and the intentional communities movement of the late 1960s and early 1970s to come into their own. When they did, the result was a number of real-life experimental communities inspired by Skinner's novel. As American Studies scholar Hilke Kuhlmann has noted in her assessment of Walden Two–type communities, 'In the late sixties and early seventies, thousands of young people refused to follow the beaten path and set out to form intentional communities. With the heyday of behaviorism and communal living coinciding, it is perhaps not astonishing that *Walden Two* inspired some readers to try out Skinner's concept of the good life' (Kuhlmann, 2005, p. x).

As Morawski (1982) has argued, psychologists' utopias provide valuable material with which to explore the interplay between psychology and society, and provide an opportunity to consider psychology both 'as a knowledge system *and* as a social instrument' (p. 1083). In the case of *Walden Two* and the communities it inspired, we have the unique opportunity to evaluate Skinner's utopianism not only as a literary or theoretical product, but as an exercise in real-life social practice (Kuhlmann, 2005). As one of the characters in Skinner's novel put it, utopianism is 'a job for research, but not the kind you can do in a university, or in a laboratory anywhere ... you've got to experiment, and *experiment with your own life!* [italics in original]' (Skinner, 1948, p. 9).

In this chapter, I document, analyze, and assess the real-world manifestations of Skinner's move from laboratory to life by closely examining two of the intentional communities that took *Walden Two* as their original inspiration. Twin Oaks, located in the lush countryside of central Virginia, provides a living, growing, and working example of one group's attempts to 'live the dream' inspired by *Walden Two* (see Komar, 1983). Los Horcones, in the arid desert of Sonora, Mexico, is a community whose dedication to applied behavior analysis has been instrumental in creating a version of the good life that promotes egalitarianism, cooperation, and pacifism.

Psychologists have frequently been criticized for doing little to advance the welfare of society, and for using their science to maintain, rather than change, the status quo (see Fox, 1985; Prilleltensky, 1989). Skinner's own philosophy and the techniques arising from it have been extensively criticized on these grounds by behaviorists and non-behaviorists alike (see Holland, 1978; Lamal, 1989; Prilleltensky, 1994; Winett and Winkler, 1972). It is clear that many of these criticisms have been and continue to be valid. The observation that behavior modification has traditionally done less to change oppressive environments than to change the behavior of the individual to adapt to these environments has been a source of concern for both the proponents and critics of applied behavior analysis, as I have already shown (see also Krasner, 1962; Malagodi, 1986). However, in this chapter I propose that a reassessment of Skinner's utopianism and its real-life repercussions reveals an under-documented reformist element that is often overlooked by those who assess Skinner's legacy from a contemporary and presentist standpoint, and who use only traditional behavior modification programs as the basis for this assessment.

Skinner's legacy of utopianism and social meliorism has had a deeper impact than academic discussions of behavior modification suggest. In fact, some contemporary critics have outlined proposals for radical social change that explicitly mimic the very ideas Skinner proposed in *Walden Two* (e.g., Crowe, 1969; Fox, 1985; Sarason, 1974). According to these thinkers, the solution to the ecological and psychological problems of a capitalist, centralized state is a decentralized system of small, libertarian socialist communities in which members redevelop a sense of community and interdependence that simultaneously fosters healthy individuality. As Fox (1985) has written, '[S]ociety should be reorganized as a network of smaller groups that would encourage a sense of belonging and enhance cooperation' (p. 52). He has argued that in a centralized state, people's ability to function autonomously diminishes, and that only through decentralization would people 'eventually regain that ability as well as their motivation to protect the commons' (p. 52).

Although stated in somewhat different terms, the sentiments of these libertarian socialist writers echo what Skinner has said about the need for a return to small communities where face-to-face interaction of members and environmental accountability bring the contingencies of behavior in closer proximity to actual behavior. In Skinner's scheme, Walden Two was intended to be just one community in a plan involving

the reorganization of society into exactly such a system.[2] It is no coincidence that many of the communities inspired by Skinner's novel are
implicitly libertarian socialist or anarcho-communist, and continue to
attract members sympathetic to this orientation. As one member of
Twin Oaks has noted about his motivation in joining the community:

> In college, reading *Utopia* by Sir Thomas More convinced me that the class
> system of rich and poor is inexcusable. Someone gave me a pamphlet on
> anarchism, and after reading it I thought that it would be better to orga-
> nize society according to the principles of anarchist-communism. I read 'A
> Walden Two Experiment: The First Five Years of Twin Oaks Community' by
> Kathleen Kinkade and decided that if I was going to go around advocating
> anarchist-communism, I had better try actually living that way first. While
> not an anarchist-communist community, Twin Oaks came fairly close.
> (Nexus, personal communication, 7 July 2000)

Twin Oaks and Los Horcones: The Reality of Walden Two

The best-known efforts to apply Skinner's utopian ideals to real-life community are Twin Oaks in Virginia and Los Horcones in Sonora, Mexico.
These two communities, although extremely different, both originated
in their early founders' desires to use Skinnerian principles to change
and improve society. Los Horcones has remained ardently committed to
a way of life guided and informed by an experimental science of human
behavior. Because of this commitment, it has described itself as the only
true Walden Two community in existence. Twin Oaks, although originally inspired by the novel *Walden Two*, expanded and modified its ideological underpinnings to encompass the growing human potential
movement and to attract new members who were not themselves committed to behaviorism. The impact of Skinner and *Walden Two* at Twin
Oaks, although catalytic, is now very difficult to discern, if not completely absent.[3] I will focus on these two communities because their similarities and differences are instructive of how Skinner's behaviorism
fared when subjected to real-life application.[4] Although both were originally inspired by *Walden Two* and have come to share very similar socialist and humanistic philosophies, Twin Oaks found it necessary to move
beyond behaviorism, while Los Horcones has assimilated the science of
behavior into everyday life. If Twin Oaks is no longer behaviorist, how
can its development shed light on the impact of Skinner's utopianism
on real-world efforts to create the good life?

There are a number of reasons why Twin Oaks provides a particularly interesting focus for this analysis. It has become one of the best-known and most successful intentional communities in the United States, as judged by its stability, influence, and longevity: it was founded in 1967 and has been in continuous existence since that time. It is an active member of the Federation of Egalitarian Communities and has spawned several of the communities with whom it shares membership.[5] Most importantly, however, the community's early attempts to use *Walden Two* as a blueprint, and its ensuing successes *and* failures, provide important material with which to analyze the practicability of Skinner's ideas in a real-life social context and to assess his utopian legacy.[6] Specifically, analyzing Twin Oaks's trajectory from its behavioristic beginnings to its ideologically diverse present provides the opportunity to discover how the implementation of Skinner's technology of behavior fared when face-to-face with the values, social context, and individual lives of late twentieth-century Americans.

In this chapter, I provide a brief overview of the history of Twin Oaks (brief because it has been covered elsewhere; see Bouvard, 1975; Kinkade, 1973, 1994; Komar, 1983), focusing almost exclusively on its founding and early years. I pay particular attention to the original influence of Skinner and *Walden Two* and examine the ways in which Skinner's behavioral technology and behaviorist philosophy both helped and hindered the development of the community. Then, using Los Horcones as a counterpoint to Twin Oaks, I show how a community that has remained ideologically homogeneous with respect to the science of behavior has grown and developed. Although the two communities share many of the same social values, Los Horcones has not strayed from its commitment to the science of behavior. As a result, its development has been quite different from that of Twin Oaks, and it has had a smaller cultural impact, at least in terms of spawning other communities and attracting members. Nonetheless, the group's commitment to behavior analysis has helped them develop what they see as a true philosophy of change.

Twin Oaks: Beyond Walden Two

To comprehend what the B.F. Skinner novel *Walden Two* meant to me in the early years, you have to understand that I was in love. Not with anyone I knew, all just flawed humans, but with Frazier ... I was also in love with Frazier's creation. I longed to spend my life at Walden Two ... It had everything I wanted. (Kinkade, 1999, p. 49)

These words, written by Kat Kinkade, one of the founders of Twin Oaks, express the passion and fervor that Skinner's novel inspired for many readers in the 1960s and 1970s. I have shown in chapter 1 that many critics decried *Walden Two* as anti-humanistic, sterile, regimented, and dull. Many believed that the science of human behavior applied to real life would result in a dystopian Brave New World. However, despite these powerful objections, reaction to *Walden Two* was not uniformly negative. Coinciding with the growth of the communities movement in the late 1960s and throughout the 1970s came a growing interest in Skinner's novel. For example, a reader who was already committed to cooperative living wrote:

> I'm an Aldous Huxley fan and a humanist and therefore an automatic critic of anything smaking [*sic*] of psychological manipulation, but I must say that I have reversed my original opinion of *Walden Two* since the breaking up of our commune makes many of your suggestions painfully meaningful.[7]

One precocious and independent-minded fourteen-year-old writing to Skinner noted the widespread negative reaction to the novel, but declared his allegiance to the *Walden Two* model in the following words:

> Young as I may be (although this may be a reason) I appear to be the only one of the others I know who read your book (my two brothers, my teacher, and a friend) who does not believe the Walden society would 'belittle man' or 'turn us into robots.' In fact I suppose I could and would become a member of such a utopia as soon as I was of age.[8]

In an era characterized by a growing disillusionment with the status quo and dissatisfaction with the values and mores of mainstream society, communal living appealed to many as a potential solution to personal, ideological, and social crises. For some of these people, *Walden Two* offered the specific blueprint for such an alternative. One reader wrote to Skinner, 'I have been running away from what I do not like, but there has not seemed to be any place worth running to. I have just finished reading *Walden Two*, and … it seems to me that there *is* a place worth running to with all alacrity [italics in original].'[9]

Thus, Skinner's vision did appeal to a significant number of pioneering would-be communitarians in the late 1960s. In 1965, one such group made an initial attempt at communal living à la Walden Two by purchasing a dilapidated house in Washington, DC, which they named Walden House. In a letter to Skinner, one of the founding members wrote:

As we understand it, the novel *Walden Two* describes an experimental community whose aim is human happiness and human progress. The system for realizing this aim is the scientific method as applied to human behavior ... This is your unique contribution, for although there are now quite a few intentional communities in the United States, none are based on this premise.[10]

In this letter, Griebe, the group's leader, outlined their philosophical commitment to the *Walden Two* model, including Skinner's ideas about educational, economic, and social reform, noting, 'About a year ago, the D.C. Walden Two Committee decided that enough discussions had been held; it was time to *do* something.' Consequently, they purchased a house which served the purpose of 'introducing solid core Walden Two-ers into a representation of Walden Two life.' They ran an advertisement in the *Saturday Review* to attract like-minded devotees of the novel. When interested parties visited Walden House, however, they found 'much filth and great disorder' in a 'dirty old building in a run-down neighborhood.'[11] Evidently, much earlier reports of these conditions had filtered back to Skinner, who quickly requested that the group not associate itself with him or the novel, despite his fundamental agreement with their organizing principles. He wrote:

Certainly there is very little in the summary of your principles ... with which I would disagree ... In any case, the thing I object to is that by using 'Walden Two' you certainly suggest to people in general that I have some association with your venture. I really do not have the time or energy to find out more about what you are doing or to take any part in sponsoring anyone's effort to build a community along the lines of *Walden Two*.[12]

Despite Skinner's initial lack of endorsement, the members of Walden House persisted, published a newsletter, and met with other people interested in starting a *Walden Two* community at a conference held just outside Ann Arbor, Michigan, in the fall of 1966. The conference was attended by interested communitarians and academic psychologists alike. However, as Kat Kinkade remarked in a 1981 interview, the two groups differed dramatically in their aims:

I began to be disillusioned with psychologists even before Twin Oaks was founded. The Waldenwoods conference in which I met the other people who were to become Twin Oaks founders was sponsored by just such psychologists, and they disappointed my expectations. For one thing they planned a psychologist-king role for themselves ... Worse, they lacked the commitment even to consider starting a community with a small group and no money. (Kinkade, as cited in Komar, 1983, p. 7)

Luckily, however, by this time Walden House (which Kinkade later described as 'a dismal failure in every way' [1973, p. 26]) had attracted the attention of a member willing to put up a sum of money to buy a piece of land on which the community could re-establish itself in a rural setting. This member's contribution came at just the right time. At the 1966 conference, the group at Walden House combined efforts with a group from Atlanta – Walden Pool – and Twin Oaks was born. On 16 June 1967 a group of eight committed Walden Two-ers settled in to create Skinner's version of the good life on a rustic farm near the South Anna River outside Louisa, Virginia.

The first five years of the Twin Oaks community have been recounted in Kat Kinkade's book *A Walden Two Experiment* (1973). Here, I will focus on the community's early attempts to implement some of the ideas presented in Skinner's novel, the dilemmas and problems they encountered along the way, and the ways in which the community endeavored to solve these problems. I hope to show that although the *Walden Two* blueprint was a technically and ideologically insufficient guide to the good life, the problems encountered by these early communitarians concretely illustrate some of the obstacles a technology of behavior encountered when it moved from the abstract to the actual: from the laboratory to life.

Labor Credits and the World of Work

The idealized version of communal life must be meshed with the reality of the work to be done in a community ... In utopia, for instance, who takes out the garbage? (Kanter, 1972, p. 64)

In *Walden Two*, Skinner outlined a system whereby the needs of all members of the community would be met in exchange for each member earning a specified number of labor credits. For most tasks, one hour of labor earned one labor credit, and four hours of work per day completed all of the work in the community. Members would be free to choose their work according to their personal tastes and abilities, although Skinner advocated a combination of skilled and unskilled tasks, including a certain amount of physical labor for everyone. Work would be undertaken according to one's own schedule. In this way, work would be maximally reinforcing – people would actually feel as though they wanted to work!

To address the problem of work that was necessary but undesirable, and work that was so desirable that there would be competition for it, Skinner suggested a system of credit adjustment whereby work that no one wanted to do would earn a higher credit per hour than more desirable tasks, which would decrease in value if they appealed to a surplus of members. In this way, the reinforcement value of every job would be adjusted inversely to its desirability, ensuring that all jobs would be performed by someone more or less willingly, or at least 'reinforcingly.'

Shortly after its inception, Twin Oaks encountered the need to establish an organized labor system. After about three weeks of the members doing basically as they pleased, the call came for some rules. Consistent with their original philosophy, they turned to Skinner's Labor Credit system. They found it ideologically appealing, in part because it overturned the mainstream notion that skilled work deserves more pay and unskilled work less pay. Kinkade wrote:

> Part of the charm of this idea, which we dubbed the 'variable credit,' is that it reverses the traditional remunerative formula (that reward for work is determined by supply and demand, and therefore skilled work, however pleasant, pays more than unskilled work, however wearing or demeaning). We agreed with Bellamy and Skinner that the traditional scheme is unfair and unnecessary, and we embraced the variable credit with a fervor almost ideological. (Kinkade, 1994, p. 31)

This ideological fervor lasted about five years, during which the community experimented with multiple versions of the variable credit system. Even before adopting this system, however, early Twin Oakers had to decide on what would count as work and what would not. Would baking homemade bread be counted as work or leisure? Some tasks that members originally classified as leisure, such as picking blackberries, were reclassified as work when they became more onerous over time. But these were small problems. As the system developed, one of the primary dilemmas was how to reach consensus on the credit value of various tasks. As Kinkade described, 'It didn't work just to ask people what they thought. The lure of higher credit tended to set people into competition with each other, sometimes squabbling with each other in their rival claims ...' (Kinkade, 1994, p. 31).

For a period, the community experimented with a system whereby each member assigned the value of a task's labor credit according to their personal attitude towards the job. For example, two people might perform identical tasks, but for one the task would be worth 1.2 credits, and for the other 0.8. This system persisted for about a year, but was finally abandoned because 'there were always people who figured out how to manipulate it for their own benefit' (Kinkade, 1994, p. 31).

Ultimately, as the community grew in size, it was observed that with enough members there were virtually no tasks that someone was not willing to do. Kinkade remarked that although Skinner would have had no way of knowing this, in a group of forty or more communitarians 'there is almost no type of work that does not attract someone. When we do run across jobs that nobody wants to do, manipulating the credit does not help' (Kinkade, 1994, p. 31).

In fact, Twin Oakers soon realized that tampering with the value of labor credits often did more harm than good. At one point, more members were eager to engage in construction work than were needed (there had been a dearth of new building in the community for some time). Accordingly, the value of construction labor credits was decreased, presumably so fewer people would be interested in the job. However, a spate of downward bidding occurred in which some members offered to do construction work for no credits, or even negative credits. Finally, an arbitrary 0.8 credits per hour were assigned to the job, which meant that in order to meet quota at the time, which was about 46.5 credits weekly, the construction workers had to work 58 hours a week. Within a few days of starting the job, most members decided construction was not as much fun as it had originally seemed.

So in 1974, after years of experimenting with variations on the variable credit system, it was declared a failure, and the community decided that almost all work would earn one labor credit per hour. Members who fell into a 'labor credit hole' of more than seven months worth of work for the last twelve months were downgraded to provisional membership, at which time a secret ballot would decide whether or not they would be allowed to stay in the community. As Kinkade wrote of this practice:

What? Punishment in a Walden Two community? No, not punishment. Contingency management. The Community offers several different ways to remain in good standing ... But eventually, one way or another, we all have to do our share of the work or leave, because it is not healthy for a large part of the Community to be angry and feel ripped off. (Kinkade, 1994, p. 35)

These examples demonstrate some of the difficulties the community encountered in implementing a system of Labor Credit that was completely faithful to the Walden Two model. Skinner had not addressed questions of morale, the social and emotional implications of devaluing work by reducing labor credit value, the issue of work becoming less reinforcing over time, the role of intrinsic motivation in the credit system, and others.[13] In the laboratory of life, Skinner's system, based on a value-free technology of behavior, had to contend with the values of a growing, counterculture-era community that was committed both to its own survival and creating a viable and satisfying alternative lifestyle for its members.

Ultimately, the system that is now used at Twin Oaks for ensuring that all of the work of the community is accomplished by its members took Skinner's Labor Credit system as its original inspiration. Twin Oakers experimented with it and settled on a system that is actually not totally dissimilar from the system used in Walden Two. In creating the good life, Twin Oakers are committed to making work maximally reinforcing without compromising the community's stability. By and large, members do not have to perform work they do not like, are free to choose what kind of work they do, and can do it whenever they please. The only exception to this rule is one dishwashing shift per week that is required of all members. This general approach worked in Walden Two, and it works at Twin Oaks to this day. What Skinner did not explicitly build into his system, but what Twin Oakers know, is that for many of them labor credits are extraneous. There is a commitment to the community and to work for its own sake that is unaffected by the presence or value of labor credits. As Kinkade wrote:

> We have members who have the same intense dedication to their work that characterizes happy professionals in the competitive outside world. Their involvement is with the work itself and with the Community. The credits are beside the point ... They want to get a good hammock brochure printed, or an engine rebuilt, or a new labor system perfected ... The reinforcement comes from the finished product ... and from the appreciation of other members of the community. (Kinkade, 1973, p. 49)

Planning and Managing an Egalitarian Society

Egalitarianism among members was a fundamental precept of the society outlined in Skinner's *Walden Two*. Honorific titles, such as 'Doctor,' were abandoned, everyone did the same amount of work and had access to the same amount of resources, and men and women were considered equals. That left open the question of how to administer a society that recognized no central authority. In Skinner's scheme, a Board of Planners and Managers oversaw the running of the community. The Planners were appointed by the Managers for a ten-year term. The Managers were specialists trained to oversee various services and divisions of Walden Two, such as Nursery, Dairy, Food, Health, etc.. Any member of the community could become a Manager by going through apprenticeship and training, and, at least in theory, Planners and Managers were accorded no special or higher status in the community. The Planners, who oversaw and were responsible for the community's general wellbeing, were required to spend half of their labor credits in regular work, including physical labor. Despite the lack of democracy, the abuse of power was theoretically avoided because there was no private wealth to exploit. The happiness of the community was the sole source of the Planners' power, or as Frazier put it, 'The despot must wield his power for the good of others. If he takes any step which reduces the sum total of human happiness, his power is reduced by a like amount' (Skinner, 1948, p. 264).

In its earliest days, with only eight members, Twin Oaks tried out a system of self-government that was based on consensus, a procedure consisting of 'discussing problems and possible solutions until everybody agreed' (Kinkade, 1973, p. 52). Although there was (ironically) considerable disagreement about adopting this approach, members were persuaded to try it out 'as an experiment.' It did not last long, as it soon became clear that, in practice, this gave the power of veto to one person who might disagree with the others on any particular issue.

Members then went back to *Walden Two* for inspiration and decided on a system of Planners and Managers not unlike the system outlined in Skinner's novel. During Twin Oaks's first five years, a board of three Planners was elected to make general community decisions and oversee the running of the community. Managers were put in charge of specific areas, such as farming, dairy, child care, kitchen, construction, visitors, etc.. In the early days, there were more than enough Managerships to go around, and they were awarded based on interest and work. Decisions made by the Managers could be overruled by the Board of Planners, which itself could be overruled by the membership as whole. But, as Kinkade (1973) explained, 'such occasions are exceptional. Managers use their best judgment in making decisions that benefit the group as a whole. They have nothing to gain by doing otherwise' (p. 55). In a statement strongly reminiscent of Frazier's in *Walden Two*, Kinkade wrote of the system, 'What keeps it from becoming a dictatorship is that there is nothing to gain from being dictatorial' (p. 55).

Years later, Kinkade (1994) wrote, 'Twin Oaks uses what we call the Planner-Manager form of government. We got it straight out of *Walden Two*, and it has worked remarkably well over the years' (p. 17). Refinements to the system in the intervening years included eighteen-month staggered terms for the Planners and the creation of about seventy-five Managerships (still almost as many positions as members). Today, the Planners hold public meetings to discuss all major decisions, and there is a much-used 'Opinion and Idea' ('O and I') board where members are free to post messages and documents on any aspect of community life. The Planners often consult the 'O and I' board to see what is currently of interest to the members, as well as to learn their members' views on community issues. It is usually the case that it is harder to persuade someone to become a Planner than there are too many people for the job.

This is an overly brief and overly simplistic account of the evolution of Twin Oaks government (for more detail, see Kuhlmann, 2005, pp. 92-101). Along the way there were intense ideological struggles that shaped the fundamental nature of the community to this day, including a repudiation of behaviorism. Kinkade (1994) has described that in the early years, the shared vision of the original members generally determined the course and nature of the decisions made. Dissenters were either silenced by group disapproval or left the community. Gradually, however, these dissenters began to outnumber the 'old-timers,' and a series of intense conflicts erupted. In 1974, outside facilitators were brought in to help resolve considerable internal power struggles. The facilitators brought with them a belief in the innate right of political equality for all members, and guided the community into accepting ideological diversity as a basic premise. The result, as Kinkade (1994) reported, was that 'at that point, the Community stopped advertising itself as Walden Two related, and started including in its recruitment material that no one ideology was prominent' (p. 25). She noted that however disappointing this was to those committed to the creation of a real-life Walden Two, it was nonetheless inevitable:

We couldn't keep out people with different philosophies and goals. We needed people for sheer survival, and there weren't enough Walden Two enthusiasts to go around. We didn't have, had never had, the power to accept people's presence and their labor and deny them political influence. (Kinkade, 1994, p. 25)

Thus, in practice, the fears expressed by many who read *Walden Two* and pictured a dystopian Brave New World wherein citizens were subject to the total control of a single, central authority, were unfounded, at least as suggested by the Twin Oaks experience. They were unfounded for at least two major reasons alluded to by Kinkade. First, in order to survive in terms of sheer numbers, and to attract new members, the community was forced to give up its doctrinaire allegiance to Walden Two and to accept members with diverse and dissenting beliefs, thus effectively dissolving any unified, dogmatic ideology. Second, the style of government advocated in *Walden Two* actually did serve as an effective counter-control against exploitation and the abuse of power. When put to real-life test, Frazier's statement that reducing 'the sum total of human happiness' would effectively weaken the power of the Planners proved correct.

Child Care and Education

Central to the philosophy of life in Skinner's Walden Two was the idea that children should be raised communally. The biological relationship between parent and child was accorded no special status; it was the responsibility of the whole community to care for and raise its children, looking after not only their physical needs but their emotional needs as well. Mother love, as Frazier pointed out, was not the only source of emotional gratification in Walden Two: 'We go in for father love, too – for everybody's love – community love if you wish. Our children are treated with affection by everyone ...' (Skinner, 1948, p. 98). Children were given up by their parents to be raised in nurseries, where scientifically proven principles of child-rearing were implemented. Parents were allowed to visit as much as they wished, but were not allowed to form exclusive relationships with their children. As Frazier remarked, 'We have untied the apron strings' (Skinner, 1948, p. 142).

Education in Walden Two was less structured than in traditional systems, and was much more individualized so that children could develop their unique abilities at their own rates. Much of the learning was undertaken in the workshops, fields, and laboratories of the community. The subjects a child might study were not pre-set, but were determined by his/her interests and abilities.

At Twin Oaks, the idea of communal child-rearing was immediately appealing. Although the community was not home to very many children during its first five years, the system that emerged and was practiced between 1973 and 1984 was based on the ideas presented in Skinner's novel (Kuhlmann, 1999b). A separate children's building was constructed and named Degania after the first Israeli kibbutz (Komar, 1983). Parents were expected to forego the traditional nuclear family unit, and to give up their children to the care of the community. Child care counted as creditable labor, however, and often parents would take on child care as part of their weekly work detail. In keeping with Skinner's blueprint, parents did not exercise exclusivity over their children, nor were they given special consideration in times of decision-making. It was the prerogative of the Child Manager to make these decisions.

How did this work in practice? In the beginning – before there were very many children and before separate children's quarters were built – not very smoothly. One of the first problems encountered was the unacknowledged reality that, despite the role of the Child Manager, the parent had the ultimate say regarding the care of the child. As Kinkade (1973) reported in one situation involving the wishes of a baby's father, Pete, his daughter Maxine, and the child manager Brian:

> Pete never actually said, 'This is my child, and I will determine how she is raised,' but he might as well have. As long as Maxine was with us, no matter what title we had conferred on Brian, it was Pete who was *de facto* child manager. (P. 136)

In other situations, it was difficult for the biological parents to consent to Managerial decisions, and difficult for them to be away from their children for long lengths of time, trusting that their children would be well cared for by less experienced members of the community. One baby was raised in an air crib which some enterprising members constructed when a commercially ordered model turned out to be of sub-standard quality. However, there was no systematic or long-term use of the device. Of this period, Kinkade (1973) concluded, 'Our early experience with children simply showed us that Skinner was right, and that a controlled environment is absolutely necessary in order to demonstrate better child raising than liberal America elsewhere is doing with laissez-faire' (p. 146).

For many years after the community was more solidly established, Twin Oaks had a fairly well organized child-care system. For the purposes of the system, children were divided into three age groups, designated 'metas' (infants up to age five), 'midis' (ages five to nine) and 'megas' (ages ten to teen). Newborns lived with their parents, but the metas lived in Degania, and spent most of their time there, eating breakfast and lunch, napping, playing, and sleeping. Child-care workers (sometimes parents, but also any Twin Oaker interested in working with children) would oversee and entertain the children throughout the day for hourly labor credits. Midis lived in their own rooms or shared a room with another midi in adult residences, and found play space there or in the communal dining and meeting room. Megas had private rooms in the same building as at least one of their parents.

Education was undertaken for many years in a private cooperative school run by Twin Oaks and several members of the local community who were looking for alternatives to the public school system. The school was a success largely due to the efforts of one dedicated and enthusiastic teacher, and despite attempts to maintain the school after she left, it basically deteriorated. The community then experimented with home-schooling. This too failed, partly because children who had come to know community members as friends and equals had a hard time adjusting to the structure of schooling with these same members. Bargaining and bribery were used to encourage the children to read and do exercises, but ultimately backfired as effective motivational strategies. Finally, some children attended the local Montessori school. This became an increasingly attractive option, but one that the community could not afford without making other sacrifices. The community made no serious or prolonged attempts to use behavioral principles in education. Its educational practices reflected its ideological diversity.

Today, Twin Oaks children are educated one of three ways: at the local public school, through home-schooling in the community, or at a Montessori school. Skinner's ideas as presented in *Walden Two* have all but disappeared. As Kinkade has written:

> Our children are well cared for, appropriately educated, and generally happy, but very little of this can be attributed to the purely communal aspects of the program. The fact is that the communal child rearing experiment, as originally conceived, has failed, and we are in the process of figuring out what to put in its place. (Kinkade, 1994, p. 146)

One of the reasons cited by Kinkade for the failure of the experiment was the lack of a strong central authority figure who was respected and competent in the field of child care. For many years the community did have one such manager who worked at Degania, and during these years, the program was fairly successful. When she left, the program fell apart and the parents quarreled among themselves about appropriate standards of care and child-rearing principles. Several parents threatened to pull their children out of the program. As the system evolved, it was decided that child care would be only partly creditable, leaving as it did (especially with older children) time to do other tasks simultaneously. Parents therefore sometimes felt as though they had to work extra hard simply because they had exercised their natural right to have children. Many members object to children in the community at all, and families are asked to live apart from other members in family residences.

Komar (1983), writing during the heyday of the child program, remarked, 'Among Twin Oakers, the *Walden Two* philosophy of child care was never completely accepted nor was it ever completely rejected' (p. 202). Essentially, the program incorporated the idea of communal care, without fully abandoning the idea of a special relationship between children and their biological parents. This led Komar to conclude that, in its early years, the program offered 'the best of both worlds,' providing 'each child with an unusual amount of love and attention as well as the benefits of communal child care' (p. 199). Kinkade, however, writing at a later stage of the community's development, expressed disappointment that the raising of children at Twin Oaks had not followed Skinner's design more closely. Although acknowledging that Twin Oaks produced young people who were 'attractive, healthy, and socially precocious,' she also remarked:

> I am disappointed. This is not what I envisioned. I meant for behavioral engineering to be taken seriously. I meant for our children to learn self-control, genuine intellectual curiosity, pleasant manners, and other dazzling rarities, all before the age of 6, as *Walden Two* promised. But this was not something I could influence at any stage ... No amount of politics will prevent a parent from determining the personality of his or her child. (Kinkade, 1994, p. 141)

In summing up all of these problems, Kinkade (1994) remarked, 'Reaching agreement in community is not easy. Raising children is not easy. Reaching agreement on raising children in an egalitarian community is, so far as I can tell, impossible' (p. 152).[14]

Skinner and Twin Oaks

This brief overview of some of the areas in which Twin Oaks attempted to put *Walden Two* principles into practice illustrates the real-world difficulties of bringing the laboratory to life. Although Skinner's technology was supposedly value-free, the good life depicted in *Walden Two* was actually replete with Skinner's own social values and opinions about what the good life should look like. It was perhaps these values, more than a technology of behavior, that influenced the development of Twin Oaks. As a community, it now adheres strongly to the principles of non-violence, cooperation, and egalitarianism. All of these values were present in *Walden Two* and were consistent with Skinner's own vision, but they had little to do with his technology of behavior, per se. Nonetheless, some of Skinner's ideas did play an important role in the creation, early history, and evolution of the community. As Kinkade remarked of Skinner's influence during Twin Oaks's first formative years:

> In general our approach to systems has been to take first the ones proposed in *Walden Two* and stick to them as long as they work well. As we find fault with them, we then make changes to correct the faults and make the system fit our situation better. Skinner's book has been of immense service to us in giving us a point of general agreement for a starting place. (Kinkade, 1973, pp. 56–7)

Despite the well-documented and accurate observation that Skinner himself was little interested in setting up an actual community,[15] I would argue that Skinner *was* supportive of Twin Oaks and its efforts, even though he was not as involved as the founders would have liked. His support of the community has been underdocumented. Accounts to date have conveyed the impression that Skinner had little to do with the community (see Kuhlmann, 2005, pp. 87–8), but archival evidence indicates that Skinner was not only supportive of the Twin Oaks endeavor, but was also actively interested in the community's progress. He endorsed its members' efforts both publicly and privately, and made financial contributions to the community. Although his efforts fell short of founders' expectations, they nonetheless indicate an active interest that has typically been downplayed.

Skinner was engaged in regular correspondence during the 1970s with Kat Kinkade, David Ruth, Gerri, Chip, and Piper – five active members of Twin Oaks (some members at that time gave up their last names when they joined the community). Although he visited Twin Oaks only once, there is archival evidence that he met with Twin Oaks members in Cambridge[16] and that he invited them to lecture at Harvard.[17] In a letter to a member of the East Wind Community, which was set up by Kat Kinkade, Skinner wrote, 'My failure to go there [Twin Oaks] does not mean a rejection of their work. I have seen many people from Twin Oaks who have come to visit me here and have worked closely with Kat Kinkade in preparing a manuscript.'[18] Additionally, he maintained an active interest in the day-to-day running of the community and often offered his ideas and suggestions. For example, in one set of correspondence, he collaborated with a Twin Oaks member about the purchase of a television and video-recording equipment for the community, even offering to tape shows which might be of interest. He wrote, 'I really think this will make a difference and hold some of the people who might otherwise drift away. I hope you don't mind my meddling in the affairs of the community.'[19] In another example, in a letter to David Ruth, Skinner wrote:

> Here is an interesting copy of the *Futurist* dealing with appropriate technologies that I thought you would find useful if you have not seen it. It seems to me that the small community is ideal for developing an appropriate technology and there are lots of good ideas here.[20]

In addition to intellectual and practical exchanges, during at least one crucial point in the community's development Skinner also offered financial support for their efforts. In a 1976 report on Skinner's visit to Twin Oaks, David Ruth wrote candidly of the community's struggles with its identity and its ideology. He remarked (and I will take the liberty of quoting at length here in order to convey a sense of Skinner's attitude towards Twin Oaks):

> Now what does all of this have to do with B.F. Skinner's first visit to Twin Oaks? It's intimately related, I'll argue, because Skinner listened to us talk about most of the above ... and still he seemed genuinely impressed by our efforts. The question of course is 'Why?' If anyone would be expected to find us laughable compared to *Walden Two*, Skinner would be. It's possible, certainly, that his enthusiasm was feigned; he was, after all, almost superhumanly charming through a lunch that saw all of us juggling our dishes because we'd neglected to prepare a dining space adequate for him and the 12 others who accompanied him. He smiled even as he ate watermelon that had inadvertently been soaked in borscht, gamely declaring it to taste

good. Still, he was satisfied enough that what we've been doing has some significance that he decided to help us through our current financial difficulties with a loan of $2000.[21]

Later in this same report, Ruth recounted Skinner's observation that 'I would have been amazed if your experience in trying to build a community hadn't forced you to change some of the things that were only ideas in my head some 30 years ago.' Ruth also observed that the community's experimental attitude would certainly have met with Skinner's approval. He concluded that it was 'our willingness to work out with each other ways in which to test out the ideas of our time (his own and those of others) that impressed Skinner.' Indeed, in a letter to Gerri (a Twin Oaks member who served two years as a Planner), Skinner wrote, '[Y]ou and East Wind are not really much like *Walden Two*, nor are you like a kibbutz, but the whole point of *Walden Two* was to experiment with the good life, and you are doing that ...'[22]

Skinner, however, was critical of some aspects of Twin Oaks social practices. He was concerned that the community, in its emphasis on creating the good life for its members, would not have much impact on the wider culture. He wrote: 'Twin Oaks could be one of the great experiments of the twentieth century but if its members are merely content to seek a good way of life for themselves, that is the end.'[23] He was also dismayed that members of the community did not seem to want to experiment with alternative child-rearing and educational practices, seeing this as one of the great opportunities for social and cultural reform.

After the NOVA documentary that profiled Skinner's visit to Twin Oaks, he received dozens of requests from viewers interested in receiving information about both Twin Oaks and other Walden Two communities. Twin Oaks supplied him with information sheets, which he sent out along with their address and those of two Twin Oaks–inspired off-shoot communities, Aloe Community in North Carolina and East Wind in Missouri, as well as the address for Los Horcones. Although never a member of Twin Oaks, it is apparent that Skinner did support their efforts through personal endorsement, monetary donations, a lively interest in the day-to-day running of the community, and concern for their long-term prospects and goals.

An objective assessment of Skinner's utopian legacy must conclude that in the case of Twin Oaks, his influence was perhaps more catalytic than systematic. However, Kinkade (1994) has noted that 'without *Walden Two*, Twin Oaks would not be here' (p. 51). Remarking on their

Labor Credit system and Planner-Manager system, among other aspects of Twin Oaks life, she remarked, 'To this day, 31 years later, one can find a thick stratum of Walden Two influences throughout our community culture' (p. 51). Several other smaller communities, such as the Dande-lion Community near Kingston, Ontario, as well as Sunflower House in Lawrence, Kansas, and Sydelle House in Kalamazoo, Michigan, were all part of the 'Walden Two movement' which stretched across North America during the 1970s (Altus, Kuhlmann, and Welsh, 1999). Other communities have remained more closely dedicated to Skinnerian prin-ciples and to the science of behavior in constructing their version of the good life, and have succeeded to a modest extent. Of these, the most notable is Los Horcones in Sonora, Mexico (see Altus, 1999; Chance, 1999; Comunidad Los Horcones, 1989; Robinson, 1996).

Los Horcones: Rhetoric and Philosophy of Change

It is clear that Skinner's influence on the intentional communities movement was a significant social phenomenon, despite the changes and developments experienced by the many *Walden Two*–inspired com-munities over the years. In this section, I provide a brief overview of the history of Los Horcones to illustrate one group's commitment to using the science of behavior to radically readjust and transform traditional social practices. Unlike Twin Oaks, Los Horcones continues to be ideo-logically committed to the science of behavior. Although members do not have to be behaviorists, they do have to conform to the behavioral practices of the community. The impact of this orthodoxy on the devel-opment of the community is discussed.

The Science of Behavior in Social Practice

> I am very committed to a science of behavior. I believe that only by apply-ing this science can we design a better community ... A science of behavior, or perhaps better stated as an *appropriate* [italics in original] application of this science, can enormously contribute to our shaping of an ideal society and solving global problems. (Robinson, 1996, p. 152)

These words were written by Juan Robinson, one of the founders of Los Horcones, approximately twenty-three years into the community's exis-tence.[24] Los Horcones describes itself as a humanistic communitarian soci-ety that uses the science of behavior to design cultural and social practices consistent with this orientation. The early impetus for the community, like the impetus for many of Skinner's own writings, was the founders' concern about pervasive social problems such as hunger, war, discrimination, poverty, pollution, and injustice. From its inception, the community has been committed to using the methods of applied behavior analysis to try to address some of these problems. The founders of Los Horcones, unlike the founders of Twin Oaks, used Skinner's novel *Walden Two* as a literary reference, but never as a working model (Comunidad Los Horcones, 1982). It was the community's belief that constant experimentation and change were the keys to successful cultural design and the solution of social problems, not the specific practices outlined in Skinner's fictional utopia. Thus, it was the experimental analysis of behavior that catalyzed and continues to infuse the way of life at Los Horcones. Even from its inception, the founders of this community were imbued with a somewhat different orientation than their counterparts at Twin Oaks. This, I will later argue, has had an impact on the scope of influence achieved by Los Horcones.

The first steps in building the community were taken in 1971, when Juan Robinson, a Mexican psychologist, and his wife, Mireya Bustamente, who also trained in psychology, set up a school called the Center for Children with Behavioral Deficits in Hermosillo, Sonora, Mexico. Robinson and Bustamente were interested in using their knowledge of applied behavior analysis to help treat developmentally delayed children with behavioral problems, many of whom had been diagnosed as autistic. Teachers at the school were committed to the use of behavioral technology in the education of their students, and received consultation in the use of applied behavior methods from Dr Sidney Bijou and Dr Ivar Lovaas. As it turned out, the establishment of the school was the first step in the creation of the community that would (and does) describe itself as the only true Walden Two community in existence.

In 1973 the group decided that the only way to use behavioral methods in a systematic way to create a better society was to set up a community which would function as a cultural laboratory. Several aspiring communitarians took up the challenge, and in October of that year, Los Horcones was formally established by a group of seven people, including Juan, Mireya, and a number of other friends and teachers from the Center, on the forty-five acres on which the school had been founded, just outside Hermosillo in northern Mexico. United by a desire to extend the practice of applied behavior analysis outside the confines of the school to their daily lives and to society at large, these communitarians decided to build an experimental culture. In their words:

Back in 1973, when we founded Los Horcones, we asked ourselves: Can we use behavior analysis to design a better culture? How is a culture that really promotes and takes into account the science of behavior in its design? In order to answer these questions, we needed to build a laboratory. But the lab we needed was not a place in a building. It was an experimental space at a cultural scale. We needed a group of people who could live 24 hours in this lab for many years ... In October 1973, we started such a laboratory. (Comunidad Los Horcones, 1999e)

One of the first steps in organizing the community was to outline a code of behavior. This code was based on a strict adherence to behavioral principles of self-management. In practice, this entailed the definition of the behavioral goals of the community, a clear description of procedures and practices, the observation and measurement of the results of these behaviors, and the implementation of changes based on these results. The original behavior code has now been renamed the 'Code of Communitarian Contingencies,' which outlines not only the behaviors expected of community members, but the specific circumstances under which the behavior is expected to occur and the consequences that should maintain it in order to consider it an appropriately communitarian behavior. From the beginning, the members have been dedicated to building a community based on the principles of cooperation, equality, pacifism, income-sharing, and ecological sustainability. Individualistic behaviors were deemed incompatible with communitarian ideals. The science of behavior has been used to change mainstream social practices that circumvent these values. As they put it, 'Apply psychology to build a better society, not to adapt people to the existent society' (Comunidad Los Horcones, 1999a).

In addition to deciding on its basic precepts, the community also began to expand its physical facilities. A communal dining room and children's house were built. More houses were constructed as private quarters for individuals and couples, and a communal kitchen was established. Gardens, chicken coops, and fruit trees were added. During the first seven years, the population of the community grew from seven to twenty members, not including a constant influx of interested visitors. In 1977, Los Horcones was established as a non-profit cooperative. Three years later, the community established the Walden Two International Association, which is dedicated to disseminating information about Los Horcones and applied behavior analysis via conferences, newsletters, and workshops. It was also designed to encourage the formation of new communities committed to using the science of behavior to improve social practices.

In 1980 the community considered a physical move. In addition to needing a larger piece of land, the area they occupied had recently been rezoned to allow the nearby construction of a Ford plant. This inflated the value of their property, which they then sold at a profit. They bought 260 acres of land about fifty miles from the original community and over three years rebuilt the community's facilities. During this time, the population fluctuated between twenty and forty members. In 1996, for example, the population was thirty adults and fifteen children. In 1992 the community considered expanding into the United States and purchased a house in Tucson, Arizona. In 1993 they began a community outreach program and Special Education Center in Hermosillo. In 1999 members of the community took a 'sabbatical' and traveled to Spain to investigate the possibility of establishing a Walden Two community there with help from some communitarian friends and local behavior analysts. Another objective of the trip was to offer talks, seminars, and workshops on behavior analysis hosted by behavior analysts in various European countries.

But what does daily life look like at Los Horcones? In many ways, life at Los Horcones bears a strong resemblance to life at Twin Oaks. For example, children are raised communally, and work is organized and distributed under a similar labor system. Compared to Twin Oaks, however, Los Horcones has a significantly smaller membership (about half the number of members) and is more ideologically homogeneous. These two factors, which are probably interrelated, have affected the functioning of the community in tangible ways.

In the areas of child-rearing and education, members of Los Horcones have not faced as many ideological struggles and practical problems as their Twin Oaks counterparts, largely because there have never been more than a handful of children to raise and educate at any one time. Nevertheless, the two communities do share similar child-rearing philosophies. Both consider children to be the responsibility of the entire community. Both have separate children's quarters where children can live together and be supervised by both biological parents and community parents. In the area of education, Los Horcones has adhered more strongly to behavioral teaching methods than Twin Oaks. The community has its own school called the Study Center, where children of elementary and junior high-school ages master material presented in a format modified from Fred Keller's personalized system of instruction. This is in contrast to Twin Oaks, which does not adhere to any one teaching philosophy (for further information on child-rearing, see Comunidad Los Horcones, 1999b).[25]

At Los Horcones, labor is organized under a system similar to that used at Twin Oaks. Labor coordinators in each area (e.g., construction, bookkeeping, education, etc.) oversee the work that needs to be done and divide the time it will take to complete the work equally among the members. This results in an hourly quota of usually six to nine hours per day. The system is somewhat less complex than the system at Twin Oaks because there are fewer members. Members are encouraged to work with the coordinators in designing their work, and they are free to choose tasks they prefer and to perform a variety of tasks. In this way, work is designed to be maximally reinforcing. Because membership is low, some work must be assigned (for further information on labor, see Comunidad Los Horcones, 1999c).

Thus, child-rearing, education, and labor are conducted similarly in both communities, although Los Horcones, with its smaller membership and ideological homogeneity, seems to have had a smoother development. In the area of government, members of Los Horcones have developed a system called Personocracy.

Personocracy at Los Horcones

Los Horcones has defined their system of government, personocracy, as government 'of the people, for the people, and by the people as individual persons' (Comunidad Los Horcones, 1999d). Community members distinguish it from democracy, which is government by the majority, and from totalitarianism, which is government by few. Personocracy was developed and tested experimentally over the first nine years of the community's existence and has been implemented since 1982. As it is described, personocracy maximizes the reinforcing consequences of pro-social behavior and is non-hierarchical and cooperative. It involves every member in the decision-making process for each area of the community's functioning.

In practice, for example, each of the agriculture, construction, education, and recreation areas has its own coordinator, but anyone who wishes to can become a coordinator in new and existing areas. Additionally, all interested members participate in all decisions made in each area through open meetings. Ongoing suggestions for each area can also be made by writing them on lists posted on the community bulletin board. Individual commitments to follow through on specific decisions are also publicly recorded and monitored. Because decisions are made publicly, personocracy is called a transparent form of government. When members cannot reach a decision, decision-making is deferred until those who disagree have a chance to gather more information about their respective positions. When a decision is reached, it is posted publicly for those who were not in attendance. If anyone not present disagrees with the decision, he or she has a chance to present more information.

Another important feature of personocracy is its educational component. Anyone who wants to become a coordinator for any area is educated by the existing coordinator. Additionally, however, it is a function of government to teach and promote skills that contribute to the smooth functioning of personocracy, such as cooperative participation, problem-solving, and communitarian behaviors (Comunidad Los Horcones, 1999d).

In this form, personocracy sounds very similar to decision-making by consensus. The community distinguishes it from such, however, and views it as cooperative decision-making. Presumably, if consensus is not reached, a decision is still made. One wonders, however, how often this occurs. The members write: 'Because personocracy teaches members to effectively participate in decision making to achieve to a common benefit, in its practice at Los Horcones we have observed that agreement is rapidly achieved' (Comunidad Los Horcones, 1999d). At Los Horcones, dissenters are few as dissent is not inherently a very communitarian behavior. Kuhlmann notes that despite this non-hierarchical structure, Juan Robinson nonetheless exerts significant charisma and authority, evoking a role that is reminiscent of Frazier in Skinner's novel (Kuhlmann, 2005, p. 156).

The Unified Environment

In comparison to Twin Oaks, Los Horcones has suffered many fewer ideological crises and has followed its behavioristic path without deviation. Although its founders and members have written many papers about the practices, theories, and philosophy of the community, less has been written about the daily lives of its members, their interpersonal and social dynamics, and the community's organizational and political struggles. Thus, it appears on the surface as though Los Horcones has had comparatively fewer growing pains. Commenting on this disparity between the two communities after a visit to Los Horcones, Kinkade has remarked, 'I did not think that what made them operate so well was behaviorism … I think it's charisma; I think it's Juan' (Kinkade, as cited in Kuhlmann, 1999a, p. 39). Whether Kinkade is right, and it has been the charisma of one of the community's founders, the community's ideological homogeneity, the success of applied behavior analysis in creating an efficiently managed community, or any combination of other reasons, it is true that Los Horcones continues to operate smoothly and remains committed to disseminating the value of applied behavior analysis through workshops, presentations, teaching, and writing. But how exactly has the science of behavior been used to reform social practices at Los Horcones?

The members of Los Horcones use the concept of macrocontingencies – sets of contingencies that work together to shape and maintain behavior – to guide their work. They have observed that efforts to change behavior in many mainstream social institutions have failed because only one or a small set of contingencies is usually targeted for change. They write, 'Acting to change a contingency without changing other interrelated contingencies is like trying to change behavior without changing the environment' (Comunidad Los Horcones, 1999e, p. 3.). A related concept, called the unified environment, has directed efforts to analyze and change complex systems of macrocontingencies. The unified environment is the chain of environmental events that works together to maintain a particular behavior. As the community sees it, 'Just as there are chains of responses, there are chains of environmental events. No event in the natural environment of an organism occurs in isolation from other events. Environmental events are interrelated. We call the sum of such events the *unified environment* [italics in original]' (Comunidad Los Horcones, 1989, p. 37).

Through the practice of applied behavior analysis informed by the concept of the unified environment, the community has been led to a set of core values emphasizing cooperation, egalitarianism, non-commercialism, and non-violence. It is these values, operationalized as communitarian behaviors, that the community continues to embody and promote. It is perhaps no coincidence that the same fundamental values underlie life at Twin Oaks. Skinner's novel appealed to many communitarians of the late 1960s and early 1970s who were ready to reject the values of mainstream society. Many of these values were implicitly condemned in *Walden Two*, despite the fact that Skinner wrote the novel more than twenty years before counterculture unrest. Segal (1987) has written:

> It is remarkable that in 1948, when much of the world was just turning from war production to the frenzied production of consumer goods, Skinner had the prescience to propose a communitarian life based on respect for nature and conservation of its resources. He foresaw communal ownership of essential machinery and technological gadgetry, and a high standard of living based on nonmaterialistic values. (P. 154)

Instead of using behavioral technology to help members adapt to existing institutions and practices, the members of Los Horcones are committed to using this tool in a philosophy of change, and to creating a new experimental culture to replace the existing culture. They realize that this is a lofty goal, remarking that 'it is relatively easy to build an experimental chamber compared to building an experimental culture' (Comunidad Los Horcones, 1999e). As Juan Robinson (1996) noted of the community's achievements and ideals:

> Los Horcones should be examined and appreciated more for the possibilities of social change it represents, rather than for what we have achieved so far ... We have not yet developed a perfect communal society at Los Horcones, but radical behaviorism helps us to find our way along that difficult and challenging road. (P. 153)

Members of Twin Oaks would undoubtedly agree that they too have yet to develop a perfect communal society. The main difference between the two communities remains the early ideological diversification at Twin Oaks and the ongoing behavioristic hegemony at Los Horcones. Yet both communities began with a similar purpose – the creation of a radically new way of life – and have developed highly similar social values. It might be argued that the influence of Twin Oaks has been more secular and widespread than that of Los Horcones. It is difficult to assess whether Los Horcones's impact has been limited largely because of its strong behavioristic orientation or a combination of other reasons, including its geographic location. The community is physically, as well as philosophically, removed from mainstream American society. Unlike Twin Oaks, it has achieved recognition largely within academic circles. The long-term impact of both communities, however, may be a far less tangible one than membership rosters and magazine articles can convey. Their very presence serves as a reminder that utopian speculation, no matter how idealistic, is necessary for any chance at widespread social transformation. As Moos and Brownstein (1977) have put it, it is only when this speculation occurs that 'the long and difficult undertaking of defining the content of a new society can begin' (p. 277).

Skinner's Utopian Legacy

Utopian writing is never pure fiction. It usually contains just enough of an element of truth so as to seem, tantalizingly, *almost* within grasp. As

Kumar puts it, 'Utopia's value lies not in its relation to present practice but in its relation to a possible future. Its "practical" use is to overstep the immediate reality to depict a condition whose clear desirability draws on us like a magnet' (Kumar, 1991, p. 3). Utopias are part social and political philosophy, part literary imagination, and part wishful thinking – positively transforming the most undesirable and destructive features of the present world. As such, utopian writers comment not only on how theory can be put into practice, but also on how we may solve many of our most pressing social problems.

Skinner's utopian legacy is most clearly represented in the efforts of those individuals who in the late 1960s and early 1970s found enough inspiration in *Walden Two* to radically change the way they lived their lives. Whether the influence of behaviorism was largely catalytic, as at Twin Oaks, or whether it continues to significantly affect both social values and cultural practices, as at Los Horcones, Skinner's legacy was profound. *Walden Two*, like any good utopia, held out the promise of a dream while making it seem almost a reality. It was this near-reality that inspired a generation of highly disillusioned young Americans in the late 1960s. As Komar (1983) remarked:

> The mere fact that Skinner broke ground for *Walden Two* in the American here and now, provided a solidifying start. Moreover, he reinstated the high value of some of America's best qualities: organizational skill and handyman practicality; the patience and perseverance – by God – to make things work. The fevered protest of the sixties cried out for this cool treatment. (P. 10)

Thus, it was a potent mixture of Skinner's practical guidelines and powerful utopian strivings that conspired to bring the *Walden Two* vision to reality. As Kat Kinkade concluded several decades into living the dream, 'For me and for Twin Oaks, the vision of *Walden Two* has died, but when it was alive it did good things! Thank you, Skinner, for writing the book that inspired us' (Kinkade, 1999, p. 52).

Ironically, this very inspiration, which itself seems to defy behavioristic analysis, was what galvanized early Walden Two-ers into action. In transforming Walden Two into a real-life social experiment, they tore down the four walls of Skinner's box and experimented on themselves in the laboratory of life. They soon found that much more than environmental contingencies were required to make their dream a reality. However, the dream itself was a potent reinforcer:

None of the things on the scale between pellets and diamonds inspired the thousands of visitors and members who have contributed their labor to the Twin Oaks experiment over the years. These people worked and sacrificed for the sake of a dream. It may not be possible to verify those dreams in the reductionist terms governing a mechanistic behaviorist laboratory; nonetheless, the men and women in this social experiment dropped the pellets. It was the dream they carried, and thus far, the dream has carried them. (Komar, 1983, p. 62)

Conclusion: From Laboratory to Life

A third Baconian theme completes the story. The New Atlantis *was the first utopia I read. A better world was possible, but it would not come about by accident. It must be planned and built, and with the help of science ... By its very nature an experimental analysis of behavior spawns a technology because it points to conditions which can be changed to change behavior. I said as much in my own* New Atlantis, Walden Two.

Skinner, 1983a, p. 412

Science and technology have always been closely interwoven. Practical problems usually come first and their solutions are then taken over by a basic science ... But there are contributions in the other direction as the methods and results of scientific research come to be applied to practical affairs ... In the long run, the distinction between basic and applied science is probably not worth maintaining.

Skinner, 2004/1968, p. 207

One could easily argue that this account of the history of Skinner's technology of behavior ends prematurely, at the climax of the story rather than the dénouement. The decade of the 1970s saw the publication of *Beyond Freedom and Dignity* (Skinner, 1971a) and Skinner's rapid ascent to the status of public intellectual; it saw the heyday of the intentional communities movement, in which *Walden Two* played an important, if not sustained, role; it saw the rise of the self-help through self-control genre that I described in chapter 5; and it saw the rapid professionalization of behavior analysis coincident with increasing public awareness of a distinct brand of behavioral engineer: the applied behavior analyst (see Goodall, 1972).

As I have shown, however, the 1970s was also a period in which limits were placed on behavior analysts' sphere of activities and influence; a period in which scientists generally, and behavior modifiers specifically, were reigned in, called to accountability, and forced to confront issues of ethics, values, and professional identity. It was the period during which Skinner's ideas were tried out most enthusiastically in the laboratory of life. In a sense, the 1970s was the decade in which behavior analysis grew from a gawky adolescent full of unrestrained idealism, to a young adult cognizant of the responsibilities of increased maturity and influence. As the father of the child, Skinner, although proud of his progeny's accomplishments, was himself growing somewhat disillusioned about the future of the world and the role a technology of behavior might play in improving it. *Beyond Freedom and Dignity,* for all of its behaviorist polemic, can be read as an impassioned plea by an aging scientist not to let the world go to hell in a hand basket. Skinner would live for another nineteen years, however, and would witness many more changes, both encouraging and discouraging, in both the field he fathered and society at large.

In this concluding chapter, I attempt to provide a dénouement of sorts by answering, at least briefly, the following three questions: What happened to the behavior modifiers? Where and in what forms does Skinner's technology of behavior persist now? Why have I characterized it as his enduring cultural legacy?

What Happened to the Behavior Modifiers?

By the early 1970s, behavior analysis had already passed a number of milestones of professionalization. In 1958 the *Journal of the Experimental Analysis of Behavior* (*JEAB*) began publication as an outlet for basic research in the operant tradition, and in 1964, Division 25 of the American Psychological Association (APA), devoted to the experimental analysis of behavior, was formed. One catalyst for both the journal and the division (virtually the same group of people founded both) was the perception that operant research was not being given a fair hearing in other journals or in the APA convention program. For these scientists, establishing their own journal, and then their own division with its own convention programming, were deemed partial solutions to this problem (Todd, 1996). A few years later, due to the rapid growth of the applied branch and the perception that the editors of *JEAB* were not facilitating the publication of applied studies (Wolf, 1993), the *Journal of Applied Behavior Analysis* (*JABA*) was established. Within one year of the first issue, *JABA*'s subscription rate was at about 4,300. By 1979 this number had risen to a peak of about

6,300 (Laties and Mace, 1993). However, despite an APA division and two journals, there was no independent professional organization for researchers or practitioners of behavior analysis.

By the early 1970s, the midwestern United States had become a stronghold of behavior analysis. But here again, many behavior analysts felt that their papers were being summarily rejected by the program chairs of the major academic meeting of this region, the Midwestern Psychological Association (MPA). Accordingly, in 1974, Israel Goldiamond and his colleague Gerald Mertens quickly organized an alternative two-day conference at the University of Chicago that ran concurrently with MPA. About a hundred people took part, and the group was christened the Midwestern Association for Behavior Analysis (Peterson, 1978). Planning quickly ensued to organize the next meeting, which was ultimately held across the street from MPA, at the Blackstone Hotel in Chicago in the summer of 1975. Incredibly, 1,100 people attended. The transition from a regional group to a national one was the next logical step, and the Association for Behavior Analysis was born. It continues to this day as the Association for Behavior Analysis International and houses experimentalists, technicians, philosophers, and teachers of behavior analysis alike. The major growth in the organization, however, has been in its applied branches.

In 2002 the Association moved from its university location into its own offices housing both paid and volunteer staff in Kalamazoo, Michigan. According to their Web site (see http://www.abainternational.org/chapters.asp), they have sixty-four affiliated chapters throughout the world, with 5,800 members in affiliated chapters in the United States, and 7,700 more members in non-U.S. chapters across thirty countries. A recent newsletter included updates from a number of these international affiliates, including ABA of Brazil, ABA Colombia, ABA Espana, ABA India, Israel ABA, Korean ABA, New Zealand ABA, Philippine ABA, Polish ABA, and Taiwan ABA ('Updates from ABA's Affiliated Chapters,' 2007).

Although behavior analysis, by this account, is alive and well and living in Kalamazoo (among many other places), the fact remains that despite a flourishing scientific and professional organization and a stable of journals, including not only *JEAB* and *JABA*, but *Behavior Analyst, Behavior and Philosophy, Analysis of Verbal Behavior, Behavior and Social Issues*, and *Journal of Organizational Behavior Management* (as well as European and Japanese journals of behavior analysis), it has largely removed itself from mainstream academic psychology, and any early efforts to influence the mainstream or integrate into it have largely been abandoned. As early as 1972, one author noted that operant psychology had become isolated from non-operant psychology and was increasingly insular and cult-like (Krantz, 1972). This last point was supported by the sentiments of one outside observer, who remarked: 'Not since J.B. Watson's time has any band of behaviorists seemed so assertive in its likes and dislikes and so convinced that its techniques and experimental approach will not only change psychology, but in the process reshape the world' (as quoted in Krantz, 1972, p. 95). This characterization does indeed seem to capture the crusading spirit that seized many behavior modifiers in the 1960s and 1970s, especially their belief that their system, unlike any other, had the potential to change the world.

There are certainly aspects of this 1972 analysis that remain as true today as they were over thirty years ago. Behavior analysis continues to be fairly isolated from mainstream psychology. Skinnerians publish in their own journals, attend their own conferences, and train their own students in certain remaining behavior analytic strongholds such as Western Michigan University, the University of South Florida, the University of Kansas, and the University of North Texas, among others. Behavior analysts, both experimental and applied, continue to use a specialized language that both sets them apart from other psychologists and creates a sense of in-group cohesion that is palpable at any meetings where Skinnerians predominate. In 1998, in recognition of the growing importance of applied behavior analysis in the treatment of autism and other developmental disorders and the need for control over practitioner training, a national Behavior Analyst Certification Board was established. This was the culmination of a process that began, arguably, with the Drake Conference described in chapter 4, but certainly with certification efforts within the state of Florida that began in the mid-1980s (Shook and Neisworth, 2005). It represents the completion of the professionalization process that began when the first 'behavior shapers' began reinforcing desirable behaviors in the late 1950s.

Some behavior analysts are concerned about their isolation from mainstream psychology and feel that their ability to enact widespread change is limited because of their marginalization. Some feel that cultural resistance to the philosophy underlying behavior analysis has gotten in the way of its impact, but that if behavior analysts keep working, they will eventually minimize this resistance. As Bijou has noted, 'Institutional practices are slow to change, particularly when the assumption or philosophy underlying a practice conflicts with that of a culture ... This state of affairs means that behavior analysts have to keep working hard at their basic and applied research, ... showing the general public that applied behavior analysis works better than most general practices' (in Wesolowski, 2002, p. 23).

Other behavior analysts are not bothered by the field's isolation from other areas of psychology, and are confident that the successes of behavior analysis will ultimately ensure its longevity as a perspective. As Jack Michael has noted:

> My attitude towards the whole thing is that I'm not particularly into trying to effect liaisons with other areas ... I have not spent much time and have not really wanted to see that as a problem, and I'm not trying to solve it. I think the truth will out. My attitude is, look what's happening in autism ... And in the area of neuropsychology, the neurosciences, biological orientation ..., I guess what you could say is this: I'm such an orthodox Skinnerian that I don't see changes from that perspective as having any particular value. In other words, we're doing fine. (Michael, 2004, interview with author)

As for the conviction that behavior analysis will reshape the world, many behavior analysts ardently hold to the belief that the technology of behavior could create widespread social change if only people could be persuaded to implement it on a large scale. But therein lies the paradox: if behavior analysts are experts at behavior change, why have they not been able to enact the most powerful change of all? Why have they not made behavior modifiers out of all of us?

Strongholds of the Technology of Behavior

Although Skinner's technology of behavior has not overtly changed the world in which most of us live, there are numerous areas in which applied behavior analysis has become highly visible. In the treatment of autism and other developmental disabilities, applied behavior analysis and its variations (e.g., early intensive behavioral intervention) have become the gold-standard treatment.[1] Operant techniques are used to address many other clinical problems, from attention deficit disorder to anxiety and depression. Parents and teachers use behavioral principles on a daily basis for child-rearing and classroom management purposes, many of which are explicitly Skinnerian. Behavior analysts have worked to develop environmental preservation projects and encourage pro-environmental behaviors.[2] One area that lies beyond the purview of this book, but where the technology of behavior has proved dramatically effective, is animal training. Although I have limited myself to applications of behavioral principles to human problems, our friends in the animal kingdom, from porpoises to dogs, have not evaded the behavior analysts' gaze.[3]

Technologists of behavior also continue to work very productively in the business and corporate world. Organizational Behavior Management, or OBM, is a burgeoning special interest group of the Association for Behavior Analysis. Skinnerians are frequently called upon to help design workplace safety programs (e.g., Geller, 2001, 2005), improve employee productivity and morale, reduce absenteeism, set up training programs, and address a host of other workplace issues as corporations tap into the expertise of behavior professionals. In the world where results count, and are counted, the technologists of behavior have a proven track record.

Obviously, the technology of behavior has proven its worth in several specialized niches and has, in these niches, become a clearly identifiable component of life beyond the laboratory. However, Skinnerians have not revolutionized psychology or reshaped the world to the extent that, at least in their early hubris, they hoped and expected to do. We are not all living lives explicitly engineered through the systematic application of operant principles. It is thus worth returning to the primary goal of this account: to explicate the processes through which a technology of behavior was manufactured and transported from the highly specialized and tightly controlled environment of the operant chamber to everyday life, and to show how both cultural openings and resistances influenced this process, providing opportunities for expansion, but also placing limits on its scope and spheres of influence.

As I have demonstrated with several examples, one of the key elements in this process was the adaptability of the physical design of the operant chamber itself. It lent itself fairly easily to modifications to suit human subjects, from children with autism, to hospitalized schizophrenics, to incarcerated criminals. It was gradually enlarged and eventually abstracted to produce a highly transportable set of techniques grounded in a philosophy of experimental control that allowed Skinnerians to conceptualize and in fact construct whole buildings, systems, and communities as Skinner boxes writ large. In chapter 2, I showed how the earliest of these human Skinner boxes were transparent examples of the powerful influence of apparatus in determining what kinds of research problems were studied, and the kind of research – and results – that ensued. For Charles Ferster, for example, the Skinner box was not simply a piece of apparatus, it actually was his research program. Lindsley was similarly devoted to the operant chamber, and ended up designing rooms that could record much more than a simple lever pull. In Bijou's case, although initially skeptical of 'a systematic laboratory approach,' he quickly abandoned naturalistic methods in favor of the operant chamber. In conducting their research inside the human Skinner box, all three men implicitly embraced the reductionism and determinism that Skinner's philosophy of science demanded and that was physically represented by the box itself.

Thus, as I demonstrated most clearly in chapter 5, behavioral technologists exploited the laboratory as truth spot in order to claim the universality of their techniques despite the fact that they derived from a very specific location, and were grounded in fairly restrictive assumptions about human nature. However, they were able to transport this set of techniques, if not the assumptions, to a wide and highly various range of settings, and adapted their practices to new local contexts and problems. Thus, theirs was a two-pronged approach: insist on the universality of the principles by referring to them as laws of behavior applicable everywhere and across species; and demonstrate this universality by transporting a standardized set of practices to a variety of different local contexts – for example, the mobile child study laboratory, the prison cellblock, the self-help manual. As application spread across multiple sites involving many kinds of problems and people, Skinnerian psychologists were able to blur the line between laboratory and life.[4]

To further analyze this migration, I return to the case of Ayllon and Azrin's token economy to treat institutionalized schizophrenic patients in the 1960s. It is clear that the cultural opening for the token economy was a receptivity to new treatments in the face of desperation over what to do with patients for whom antipsychotics did not work, psychoanalysis was patently inappropriate, and de-institutionalization was out of the question. The token economy represented a practical, can-do approach that was welcomed, and subsequently flourished. However, as the 1970s unfolded, the growing public perception that behavior modification was inhumane, the momentum of the patients' rights movement, and an increasing number of legal cases and decisions that influenced how psychiatric patients could be treated, slowed the development of token economies until they all but disappeared. Practical problems also played a role. Token economies were expensive to run, required staff cooperation, and were perceived as tedious to operate and monitor. Interestingly, although scientific evaluations of the effectiveness of the token economy compared to other forms of treatment were largely equivocal, it was actually in the aftermath of a monumental and highly rigorous study indicating their *superiority* over other forms of treatment (Paul and Lentz, 1977) that token economies began their precipitous decline.

In the case of the prison work I describe in chapter 4, a social willingness to try new methods of rehabilitation provided a cultural opening for behavior analysts to try out their techniques in the penal system. Again, however, push-back in the form of legal challenges to prisoners' involuntary participation in behavior modification programs, mounting concern over the ethical treatment of human subjects in behavioral research, and a shift in the balance of opinion favoring retribution over rehabilitation all served to control the work of the controllers.

Finally, in my discussion of the be-your-own-behavior-modifier literature, the American public's long-standing and vigorous appetite for self-help literature provided behavior analysts with a ready cultural opening for their approach. A staunch belief in the possibility and value of self-improvement has long been a deeply held American value. The be-your-own-behavior-modifier movement fit hand-in-glove with this ethos – almost. To decrease resistance to their approach, behavior modifiers had to overcome the emphasis on the role of *willpower* and introduce instead the importance of self-control, subtly eliding willpower with control and conveniently leaving the self undefined. In a practical move, behavior modifiers overlooked the inconsistency between a philosophy that demanded the renunciation of human agency and a technology that required human agency in order that it be adopted in the first place. To exert self-control through the careful auto-construction of environmental contingencies demanded that the agent of control commit to, decide upon, and set up those contingencies to set the whole process in motion. Thus, the be-your-own-behavior-modifier genre allowed agency back into the Skinnerian model without explicitly commenting on its presence.

In the case of Walden Two–inspired intentional communities such as Twin Oaks and Los Horcones, an impassioned commitment to alternative living and the conviction that individuals *can* enact social change were and are what propel them forward. At Twin Oaks, the ideological hegemony of behaviorism was quickly dispensed with, while at Los Horcones behavior analysis continues to offer practical guidance in living and a shared philosophical commitment that maintains the cohesion of the community.

The Technology of Behavior as a Form of Psychological Expertise

My premise from the outset has been that Skinner's most enduring cultural legacy is his technology of behavior, rather than his experimental science or his philosophy of radical behaviorism. I have outlined the historical evolution of this technology of behavior by presenting and discussing several of the projects undertaken by behavioral engineers from the 1950s through the 1970s. More than any specific finding, technique, publication, or program, however, I would argue that it was the thoroughgoing insistence on treating human behavior change like any other technological problem, and envisioning the world as nothing more, *and nothing less*, than a very large, and very elaborate, Skinner box, that stands as the most enduring cultural artifact of the technology of behavior. There have been and continue to be countless ideas promoted by countless authors on how to change behavior, but it was by talking and writing about a set of behavior change practices as a *technology* and claiming this technology as a form of expertise, that Skinnerians have made one of their most indelible cultural marks.[5] As I have shown, this technology reified a form of psychological expertise to which twentieth-century Americans were particularly receptive, although not passively so.

Rose (1992) has defined expertise as 'a particular kind of social *authority*, characteristically deployed around *problems*, ... grounded in a claim to *truth*, asserting technical *efficacy*, and avowing *humane* ethical virtues' (p. 356, italics in original). He has pointed out how the notion of expertise allows us to analyze the processes whereby psychology has been successful in infusing social reality, and in particular why it has been so successful in the liberal democracies of the West. Ward (2002) has argued that psychology has become such a highly appealing knowledge form, especially in the United States, not because it adheres consistently to a particular philosophy of science, or because it has created new material technologies (such as tests), but because it has established technologies of the self which provide people with 'seemingly essential strategies for managing and conducting everyday life' (p. 220). I would argue that Skinner's technology of behavior represents not only a technology of the self (paradoxically, given the ontological status of the self in Skinner's philosophy), but a form of psychological expertise *par excellence*.

Technologists of behavior made us believe that behavior itself could be calibrated with precision, that new forms of behavior could be engineered where none existed before, and that troublesome behaviors could be effectively reduced or even eliminated. As a professional group, Skinnerians were unprecedented both in providing a specialized language with which to talk about behavior, and in providing myriad practical demonstrations of how to change it. In effect, they successfully claimed and colonized a distinct area of expertise over which they had authorial control, but which could be disseminated effectively by a diverse cadre of technicians. They repeatedly asserted the technical efficacy and humane ethical virtues of their enterprise, even when the latter were attacked by outsiders. By calling their set of tools a technology, they simultaneously drew upon an existing cultural trope and brought into being a new way of thinking, feeling, and acting and reacting to oneself and others predicated on a practical, problem-solving, engineering approach to human behavior that resonated forcefully with a society that was simultaneously becoming both increasingly *psychologized* and *technologized.*

It can be, and has been, argued that in one form or another, a technology of behavior has been a part of life all along. However, by bringing behavior into the laboratory, and indeed into the operant chamber, and observing, measuring, manipulating, and graphing it, Skinnerian psychologists transformed it into a type of expertise that had significant cultural currency. Furthermore, the ethos of the technology of behavior, shorn of its problematic ontological foundations, was deeply rooted in the Progressivism of the early twentieth century and buoyed by the cresting wave of modernity as the century progressed.

Conclusion

I have argued that it is appropriate to consider Skinner's technology of behavior alongside other technologies and techniques as having played an important role in the psychologization of American culture over the course of the twentieth century. Unlike other techniques, however, such as testing and psychotherapy, the technology of behavior displayed its social control functions front and center, often using the language of control unselfconsciously, albeit not unproblematically. Unlike testing, which produced information about individuals and groups which could then be used for social control, behavior modification was applied directly to the individual. Unlike psychotherapy, behavioral technology could be used to create whole systems and total environments to which individuals were subjected. Although they attempted to legitimate and contextualize these social control functions within a rhetoric of benevolence and social meliorism, behavioral engineers nonetheless encountered significant cultural resistance to many of their attempts to spread this technology. This pushback forced Skinnerian psychologists to modify their techniques, and refashion their identities. In some cases, it became necessary to convince their audiences that changing one's behavior, and even one's life, was a process over which the self, despite Skinner's deterministic and agency-less philosophy, *could* take control.

Skinner's biographer, Daniel Bjork, has written, '[I]f the individual and the environment are the great focuses of the American experience, then Skinner urged us not only to consider them in relation to each other but to consider them *scientifically*' (Bjork, 1993, p. 212, italics in original). I would take Bjork's assessment one step further. In considering the relationship between the individual and the environment *scientifically*, Skinner and his followers also perceived the incredible power and potential appeal of a *technology* based on this science. To reiterate Skinner's point, 'In the long run, the distinction between basic and applied science is probably not worth maintaining' (Skinner, 2004/1968, p. 207). Nourished by the enduring American fascination with the shaping of the self, and a deeply held veneration for both science *and* its application, the technologists of behavior were pulled inexorably beyond the box and forcefully envisioned how to bring the laboratory to life.

Notes

Archival Collections Consulted

Division 25 Papers, Archives of the History of American Psychology (abbreviated
    in all endnotes as AHAP)
Division 26 Papers, Archives of the American Psychological Association
Charles Ferster Collection, American University Archives
Charles Ferster Papers, Archives of the History of American Psychology
J.V. McConnell Papers, Archives of the History of American Psychology
Metropolitan State Hospital Records, Massachusetts State Archives
B.F. Skinner Gift, Archives of the History of American Psychology
B.F. Skinner Papers, Harvard University Archives (abbreviated in all endnotes
    as HUA)
Stephanie Stolz Papers, Archives of the History of American Psychology
William Verplanck Papers, Archives of the History of American Psychology

Interviews Conducted

Teodoro Ayllon
Scott Geller
James Holland
Ogden Lindsley
Jackson Marr
Jack Michael
Edward Morris
Joseph Morrow
Joseph Pear
Julie Skinner Vargas

Introduction: Beyond the Box

1 For those unfamiliar with *Beyond Freedom and Dignity,* Skinner basically argued that since all behavior is controlled by environmental contingencies, free will is an illusion. Further, he insisted that we must give up our anti-quated and sentimental belief in autonomous man and deliberately manipu-late these contingencies to ensure the survival of the culture. Interestingly, the very first chapter of the book is entitled 'A Technology of Behavior' and begins with a plea for using a technology of *human* behavior to solve many of the problems created by unchecked physical technologies.

2 B. Wascenacht to B.F. Skinner, 10 September 1971, Skinner Papers, HUG FP 60.20, Box 9, Folder: Psychology Today replies, HUA.

3 Curtiss Ewing to the Editors of *Psychology Today,* 16 August 1971, Skinner Papers, HUG FP 60.20, Box 9, Folder: Psychology Today replies, HUA.

4 Skinner's penchant for gadgeteering and inventing is nicely discussed in Daniel Bjork's *B.F. Skinner: A Life,* the only major biography of Skinner pub-lished to date. Bjork provides a remarkably judicious, well-researched, and engagingly written analysis of Skinner's life and work, emphasizing Skinner's role as social inventor and positioning his social philosophy vis à vis several traditions in American social and political thought throughout the course of the twentieth century. Daniel Wiener, a clinical psychologist, has published a comparatively shorter psycho-biographic account of Skinner's development (see Wiener, 1996). Marc Richelle, at the University of Liège in Belgium, has written a semi-biographic account that focuses largely on correcting misper-ceptions of Skinner's work, and is rather dismissive of behavior analysis more generally. As he puts it, 'This book is about Skinner, not about the Skinnerians. The difference is an important one, since most of the controversies sur-rounding Skinner involve a permanent confusion between the two' (Richelle, 1993, p. x). Skinner's three-volume autobiography, the last volume of which was published seven years before he died, also provides a window on how a behaviorist viewed himself (see Skinner, 1976, 1979, 1983a). Finally, for a meticulously researched bibliography of the primary source works of B.F. Skinner, see Morris and Smith, 2003.

5 There have been a small number of chapters (e.g., Kazdin, 1982; Krasner, 1990) and one book (Kazdin, 1978) on the history of behavior modifica-tion. These have almost without exception been written by participants in the field and provide descriptive, uncritical, and internalist overviews. John Mills's book *Control: A History of Behavioral Psychology* (1998) offers one chap-ter on behavior modification. In contrast to the internalist accounts already mentioned, Mills is extremely critical of behavior modification and

Skinnerian psychology generally, concluding that the demise of token economies and (what he sees as) the failure of behavioral therapies disproves the theoretical basis of behaviorism. He also sees behaviorism as a form of scientistic ideology, a point I would not necessarily contest. An edited volume by O'Donohue, Henderson, Hayes, Fisher, and Hayes (2001) contains autobiographical chapters by several notable behavior analysts, many of whom did applied work, including Sidney Bijou, Ogden Lindsley, Todd Risley, Donald Baer, and others. John O'Donnell's book *The Origins of Behaviorism: American Psychology, 1870–1920* (1985) must be considered the classic historical work on the emergence of behaviorism in its intellectual, disciplinary, and social contexts, but as the time frame indicated in the title suggests, it stops short of covering Skinnerian behaviorism or behavior modification.

6 Although Skinner did write extensively about his system's application to human affairs, perhaps most notably in his 1953 book *Science and Human Behavior*, he did not actually carry out the extensions himself. This he left primarily to the cadre of applied Skinnerian psychologists who eventually became known as applied behavior analysts, or more colloquially, behavior modifiers.

7 There have been a number of useful, if non-systematic, approaches to situating B.F. Skinner and some aspects of his work in the American context. The most useful for my work has been Smith and Woodward's excellent edited volume *B.F. Skinner and Behaviorism in American Culture* (1996). More recently, Hilke Kuhlmann, an American studies scholar, has published the first non-participant account of the real-life communities that took *Walden Two*, Skinner's 1948 utopian novel, as their inspiration. She includes the transcripts of a number of interviews she conducted with community members at the end of the book (see Kuhlmann, 2005). The title of Rebecca Lemov's recent volume, *World as Laboratory: Experiments with Mice, Mazes, and Men*, suggests that Skinner and behavior modification might be covered in her account, but she mentions Skinner only in passing despite noting that he (as well as behaviorist John B. Watson) 'served as the public face of his discipline' and would not 'have been out of place in a *New Yorker* profile' (Lemov, 2005, p. 79). Finally, in her somewhat more journalistic and sensational account, Lauren Slater includes a short chapter on Skinner in her book *Opening Skinner's Box: Great Psychological Experiments of the Twentieth Century* (2004). Although the accuracy of the details of her account can certainly be questioned (see Weizmann, 2005), she does comment on Skinner's importance in changing how we understand behavior.

8 Radical behaviorism is the philosophy of Skinner's science of behavior. It opposes the position that behavior is caused by the activity, will, or function of the mind. However, unlike methodological behaviorism, which simply places

the mind out of bounds as an appropriate object of scientific study, radical behaviorism dramatically reconceptualizes the 'mental' as the realm of private events consisting of the physiological sensations of the world within the skin or the experience of the physical sensations of the body. Thus, it radically reinterprets the nature of the mind or the mental instead of simply ruling them outside the acceptable scope of scientific inquiry. Skinner viewed the private events of the world within the skin as having essentially the same ontological status as publicly verifiable events. They thus hold no unique causal status, and are equally admissible to experimental analysis, although they are, admittedly, more difficult to study. As Delprato and Midgley (1992) point out, language, thinking, and consciousness all come under the purview of the experimental analysis of behavior, but they are radically reconceptualized as forms of behavior ultimately dependent on the external or social environment for their development.

9 See Smith, 1992, for a cogent analysis of Skinner's relationship to the American technological imperative, and Smith, 1996b, for an overview of Skinner's place in American culture.

10 In an address to the Department of Psychology at Wayne State University in 1968, Skinner was asked to speak on the topic 'Psychology in the Year 2000.' In the opening paragraph of his speech, he conjectured, 'Will new drugs be discovered that will increase intelligence, control our emotions, heighten awareness, or cure psychoses? Will geneticists solve these problems through direct manipulation of the germ plasm, or will electrophysiologists do it by brain stimulation?' (reprinted as Skinner, 2004, p. 207). He concluded that although advances were assured, revolutions were unlikely and psychology in the year 2000 was more likely to comprise 'a rather conservative extrapolation of what is going on now' (p. 207). Readers can forgive him for his lack of prescience in the fields of pharmacology and genetics.

11 Recently, in the house journal of the Association for Behavior Analysis, *Behavior Analyst*, there appeared two articles revisiting the impact and nature of Chomsky's review. The first (Virués-Ortega, 2006) consists mainly of an interview with Chomsky, conducted by the author of the article in 2004, and then continued by e-mail through 2005. It provides an interesting window on Chomsky's position (which unsurprisingly remains largely unchanged), but also on his view of behaviorism, almost fifty years after the review was published. The second article (Palmer, 2006) reinforces behavior analysts' continued dislike of Chomsky and their refusal to see his critique as anything other than a complete misunderstanding of Skinner's position. This recent re-exploration of an undeniably important episode in the history of psychology stands as interesting grist for the mill for sociologists of science.

12 See, for example, Cushman, 1995, for the cultural role of psychotherapy, and Rose, 1996, for the role of the 'psy' disciplines in shaping the psychological self.

13 Recent examples of externalist histories which examine psychology's embeddedness in and influence on American culture include Ellen Herman's *The Romance of American Psychology* (1995), James Capshew's *Psychologists on the March* (1999), and sociologist Steven Ward's *Modernizing the Mind: Psychological Knowledge and the Remaking of Society* (2002). Although all are extremely useful in tracing the rise of psychological expertise in the twentieth century, none devotes extended discussion to the role of Skinner's technology of behavior in the cultural impact of psychology or to the technology of behavior as a form of psychological expertise.

14 Much of this scholarship focuses on the products and processes of the physical and natural sciences. One notable exception is Danziger's work, particularly *Constructing the Subject: Historical Origins of Psychological Research* (1990), which illuminates how the investigative practices and corresponding knowledge products of psychology have been historically and socially constituted through the relational configurations of experimenters and subjects, and addresses more cursorily how laboratory-generated knowledge is transmitted into the social world. Although the laboratory itself has been discussed in terms of its professional significance for the construction and maintenance of psychology's scientific identity (see Capshew, 1992), somewhat less has been done within the sociology of science framework to analyze whether the processes of transfer and transformation of laboratory-generated *psychological* knowledge to the outside world are similar to the processes involved in transferring knowledge about the physical or natural world.

15 Although Skinner was supportive of the development and growth of applied behavior analysis as a sub-field, he was not directly involved in it himself, as noted above. See Morris, Smith, and Altus, 2005, for an analysis of Skinner's relation to the applied branch of his system.

16 See Kantor, 1968, for a review of six distinct periods of behaviorism; see Schneider and Morris, 1987, for a history of the term 'radical behaviorism'; and see Ruiz, 1995, for a clarification of the relationship between radical behaviorism and other forms of behaviorism as grounds for a feminist reconstruction.

1: A Visible Scientist: B.F. Skinner as Public Intellectual

1 Skinner also withdrew from the programmed instruction and teaching machine enterprise around this time, preferring to leave this work to his colleagues and students while he focused on writing.

2 Other visible scientists included Margaret Mead, Linus Pauling, Barry Commoner, Isaac Asimov, Noam Chomsky, and William Shockley. However, Skinner topped the list with 82 per cent of students surveyed correctly identifying him. See also Blakeslee, 1975, and 'What Makes a Researcher "Good Copy,"' 1975.

3 See La Follette, 1990, for a review of popular stereotypes of science and scientists.

4 Capshew (1996) has argued convincingly that the Second World War catalyzed Skinner's transformation from scientific purist to behavioral engineer. He points to Project Pigeon, Skinner's Second World War development of a pigeon-guided missile system, as his first application of behavioral science to human problems (see also Skinner, 1960). But since Project Pigeon remained classified for more than a decade following the war, the air crib was the first of Skinner's ventures that received widespread popular attention. Skinner himself has remarked that his utopian novel *Walden Two* was the first time he applied scientific principles to the problems of human behavior, but although he wrote it around the same time he invented the baby box, it wasn't published until 1948. Thus, I consider the air crib his first publicly significant venture beyond the box.

5 For more information on the air crib, see Benjamin and Neilsen-Gammon, 1999. For an account of the Skinners' approach to parenting, which also includes a description of the air crib, see Jordan, 1996.

6 'Heir Conditioner,' *Industrial Bulletin of Arthur D. Little Inc., Chemists-Engineers,* no. 217, January 1946, Skinner Papers, HUG FP 60.20, Box 3, Folder: Baby Box, HUA.

7 See, for example, 'Baby Box,' 1947; 'Boxes for Babies,' 1947; 'Box-Reared Babies,' 1954; 'Heated, Air-Conditioned "Baby Box,"' 1948; 'How a Tech Professor Raises His Youngsters,' 1954; Schur, 1946.

8 As cultural historian Karal Marling has pointed out, in the 1950s the United States bought three-quarters of all the household appliances produced in the world (Marling, 1994).

9 Unsigned letter to B.F. Skinner, 30 September 1945, Skinner Papers, HUG FP 60.10, Box 1, Folder 4: Correspondence, 1928–48, HUA.

10 N. McKean to B.F. Skinner, 29 September 1945, Skinner Papers, HUG FP 60.10, Box 1, Folder 4: Correspondence, 1928–48, HUA.

11 'Carters' Box-Bred Babies Grow Healthy, Contented,' *Viewpoints,* vol. 4, no. 1, January 1964, a monthly bulletin for members of Francis I. Dupont and Co., Skinner Papers, HUG FP 60.20, Box 3, Folder: Baby Box, HUA.

12 See Benjamin, 1988, Bjork, 1993, pp. 167–90, Skinner, 1983a, and Vargas and Vargas, 1996, for more information about the history of the teaching machine and Skinner's development of programmed instruction.

13 For accounts of his attempts, see Benjamin and Nielsen-Gammon, 1999; Bjork, 1996; and Skinner, 1979. Despite the failure of mass commercial production, even sixteen years after the *Ladies Home Journal* article appeared, the baby box continued to fascinate – see Lieber, 1962, and 'Box-Bred Babies,' 1963.

14 A few writers did pick up on this point: 'With much of the communication load ascribed to the instructional machines of the future, teachers can pay a great deal more attention to their relationships with students' (Campbell, 1967, p. 64).

15 For example, in 1964, IBM merged with Science Research Associates; in 1965, Xerox purchased American Education Publications; and in the same year, General Electric acquired Time Inc.'s General Learning Corporation (Silberman, 1966).

16 Skinner's esteem for one of his own teachers is poignantly revealed in the first volume of his autobiography, *Particulars of My Life*. Here, he described the impact of Mary Graves on his cultural, intellectual, and emotional development as a middle and upper school student in Susquehanna (see Skinner, 1976, pp. 149–55). Several years before writing his autobiography, as he prepared to dedicate his book *The Technology of Teaching* to Miss Graves, he corresponded with her niece: 'I hope to write some kind of appreciation of Miss Graves, emphasizing, in particular, how rare a person she was but even how much rarer she would be today. We simply do not have the culture from which she emerged' (B.F. Skinner to Isabel H. Graves, 7 June 1962, Skinner Papers, HUG FP 60.10, Box 6, Folder #1 of 2, Misc. 1962, HUA). And in a letter to a friend in Susquehanna: 'I want to dedicate [*The Technology of Teaching*] to Mary Graves, who was possibly the most important teacher I ever had, and who was the sort of person who will, I am sure, never be replaced by a machine' (B.F. Skinner to K. Glidden, 5 March 1962, Skinner Papers, HUG FP 60.10, Box 6, Folder #1 of 2, Misc. 1962, HUA).

17 Skinner did, of course, receive some positive feedback. As one young reader gushed: 'I am 14 years old and a great admirer of yours. I have studied your "Skinner box" and I agree with its logic completely. I also have read "BFD" and found it most interesting. I think you are one of the wisest men in America today' (Ben Ivry to B.F. Skinner, undated, Skinner Papers, HUG FP 60.20, Box 2, Folder: Autographs, HUA).

18 Although, again, there were dissenting opinions. One reader pointed out that Skinner's call for more control provided a welcome antidote to the freewheeling, anything-goes frenzy of the counterculture: '[M]any people are ready to give him a careful hearing. The nation is spaced out after a binge of anarchical personal behavior that has affected everything from the campuses to Times Square' (Dickinson, 1971, p. 4).

19 Robert Newman to B.F. Skinner, undated, Skinner Papers, HUG FP 60.10, Box 7, Folder: Misc. Corr. 1971–2, HUA.

20 H.A. Franklin to the Editor of *Psychology Today*, 2 September 1971, Skinner Papers, HUG FP 60.20, Box 9, Folder: Psychology Today replies, HUA.

21 Gilbert Aberg to the Editor of *Psychology Today*, 12 September 1971, Skinner Papers, HUG FP 60.20, Box 9, Folder: Psychology Today replies, HUA.

22 B.F. Skinner to Walt Siegel, 29 March 1972, Skinner Papers, HUG FP 60.15, Box 8, Folder: Misc. 1972–8, HUA.

23 B. Wascenacht to B.F. Skinner, 10 September 1971, Skinner Papers, HUG FP 60.20, Box 9, Folder: Psychology Today replies, HUA.

24 Curtiss Ewing to the Editors of *Psychology Today*, 16 August 1971, Skinner Papers, HUG FP 60.20, Box 9, Folder: Psychology Today replies, HUA.

25 Andrew Wallace to B.F. Skinner, 24 September 1971, Skinner Papers, HUG FP 60.10, Box 7, Folder: Misc. Corr. 1971–2, HUA.

26 B.F. Skinner to the Editor, *New York Times Book Review*, 27 October 1971, Skinner Papers, HUG FP 60.10, Box 17, Folder: N-O Correspondence, 1965–71, HUA.

27 Sid Mulder to B.F. Skinner, 28 September 1971, Skinner Papers, HUG FP 60.10, Box 7, Folder: Misc. Corr. 1971–2, HUA.

28 Barbara Porter to B.F. Skinner, 23 September 1971, Skinner Papers, HUG FP 60.10, Box 7, Folder: Misc. Corr. 1971–2, HUA.

29 B.F. Skinner to Bruno Bettelheim, 31 May 1966, Skinner Papers, HUG FP 60.10, Box 6, Folder: Misc., 1961–7, 2 of 3, HUA. Bettelheim's own theoretical biases may have been well served by repeating this rumor. He was a vocal proponent of the theory that unemotional, cold mothers were the cause of childhood autism.

30 I am not suggesting here that Skinner was cold or unemotional, only that popular caricatures highlighted these qualities.

31 B.F. Skinner to Helen Bartley, 1 August 1966, Skinner Papers, HUG FP 60.10, Box 6, Folder: Misc 1961–7, 1 of 3, HUA.

32 R. Kane to the Editor of *Psychology Today*, 9 September 1971, Skinner Papers, HUG FP 60.20, Box 9, Folder: Psychology Today replies, HUA.

2: From Pigeons to People: Constructing the Human Skinner Box

1 Letter from B.F. Skinner to Bob Bailey, 17 June 1977, Skinner Papers, HUG FP 60.10, Box 25, Folder: B [A-I] Corr. 1974–9, 1 of 3, HUA.

 2 Letter from G.W. Phelps to the Editor of *Psychology Today*, 21 September 1971, Skinner Papers, HUG FP 60.20, Box 9, Folder: Psychology Today replies, HUA.

3 The free operant method refers to 'the use of any apparatus that generates a response which takes a short time to occur and leaves the organism in the same place ready to respond again' (Ferster, 1953, p. 263). Required instrumentation for the free operant method includes a manipulandum upon which the organism operates to receive reinforcement (typical examples include a key that is pressed or a lever that is pulled); a device for recording the organism's responses; a magazine or delivery chute for delivering the reinforcer; an operant chamber in which to carry out the experiment (ideally, this would be soundproofed); and automatic programming equipment so that reinforcement schedules can be set ahead of time by the experimenter and run without supervision.

4 See also Long, Hammack, May, and Campbell, 1958; and Harold Weiner's NIMH-funded work at St Elizabeth's Hospital (Weiner, 1962, 1963).

5 In the case of goldfish, the operant chambers were water-filled plastic tubes, the operant response was swimming to interrupt a light beam, and the reinforcer was a puff of oxygenated water! (see van Sommers, 1962).

6 Letter from B.F. Skinner to Charles Ferster, 1 December 1955, Skinner Papers, HUG FP 60.7, Box 1, Folder: Ferster, C.B., HUA.

7 The Pigeon Lab, or some variation of it, ran for fifty years, from 1948 until 1998. Skinner was actively involved in the Lab until about 1962. A special section of the third issue of volume 77 of the *Journal of the Experimental Analysis of Behavior* is devoted to reminiscences of the Pigeon Staff and the historical and scientific legacy of the Lab. The history of the Lab is a fascinating topic in and of itself that is unfortunately beyond the scope of the present volume.

8 For his part, Skinner described this time with Ferster as 'a near-perfect collaboration, undoubtedly the high point in my life as a behavioral scientist' (Skinner, 1981, p. 259).

9 Letter from C.B. Ferster to B.F. Skinner, 27 November 1955, Skinner Papers, HUG FP 60.7, Box 1, Folder: Ferster, C.B., HUA.

10 Letter from C.B. Ferster to B.F. Skinner, 27 November 1955, Skinner Papers, HUG FP 60.7, Box 1, Folder: Ferster, C.B., HUA.

11 For a complete history of the Yerkes Laboratories of Primate Biology, see Dewsbury, 2006.

12 This self-designation is from a copy of his curriculum vitae found in Box M92, Folder: Chimp Expt 2, Ferster Papers, AHAP.

13 For a full description of the vending machines and other apparatus, see Ferster and DeMyer, 1961, pp. 316–17.

14 Catania (2002) has pointed out that even at the Pigeon Lab 'studies with other organisms were typically always in progress' (p. 334).

15 Annual reports from Metropolitan State Hospital indicate that starting around 1953, Boston Psychopathic Hospital forged a training affiliation with Metropolitan, which accounts for the connection between Harry Solomon and William McLaughlin, who remained superintendent of Metropolitan throughout the tenure of the Behavior Research Laboratory. The annual reports for the hospital for the years 1931–69 are held at the Massachusetts State Archives in Boston.

16 For a detailed description of the rooms, subjects, and experimental procedures, see Lindsley, 1956.

17 Letter from B.F. Skinner to Philip Sapir, 19 October 1954, Skinner Papers, HUG FP 60.10, Box 2, Folder: Misc. Corr. 1950–4, HUA.

18 Letter from Philip Sapir to B.F. Skinner, 17 November 1954, Skinner Papers, HUG FP 60.10, Box 2, Folder: Misc. Corr. 1950–4, HUA.

19 Letter from B.F. Skinner to H.C. Solomon, 29 November 1954, Skinner Papers, HUG FP 60.10, Box 2, Folder: Misc. Corr. 1950–4, HUA.

20 Lindsley also noted that with the discovery of the thalidomide cases in Europe and the United States in the late 1950s, the United States Public Health Service halted the flow of drugs that could be used in human trials. This resulted in the 'kiss of death' to the BRL's drug-screening program (Lindsley, 2001, p. 149).

21 Letter from Eileen Allen to David Clark, 10 September 1999, personal collection of David Clark; copy with the author.

22 For a photo, floor plan, and full description of the mobile child study laboratory, see Bijou, 1959.

23 Letter from W.S. Verplanck to B.F. Skinner, 18 April 1956, Verplanck Papers, Box 1969, Folder 10, AHAP.

24 Wolf received his PhD from Arizona State in 1963. The psychology department there was the first to offer a specialized program in behavioral research, theory, and application. For its brief period of existence (about eight or nine years), it was known as 'Fort Skinner in the desert' (Wolf, 2001, p. 290).

25 Letter from Eileen Allen to David Clark, 10 September 1999; copy with the author.

26 Reported by Fuller in a letter from P.R. Fuller to B.F. Skinner, 29 June 1979, Skinner Papers, HUG FP 60.10, Box 27, Folder: F (A-Z), Corr. 1974–9, 3 of 3, HUA.

3: Conditioning a Cure: Behavior Modification in the Mental Institution

1 There are a number of priority claims among behavior analysts as to who was the first to use tokens systematically. See Staats, Staats, Schutz, and Wolf, 1962, for another early account of the use of tokens to help shape reading.

2 This was not necessarily an unintentional move. Ayllon recognized the power of the nurses on the ward, and saw their allegiance as crucial to the success of his endeavors. As behavior analyst Jay Birnbrauer noted ten years later: 'When behaviorists moved from their laboratories to wards and classrooms in the latter 1950s and early 1960s, it was considered crucial to secure administrative support and to work on problems that the staff (nurses, teachers, etc.) found most distressing' (Birnbrauer, 1978, p. 176). Interestingly, from the point of view of the framework of this book, later in this same article he wrote, 'Entry into those settings itself was a result of our seeking controlled environments that were much like the animal and human operant chambers with which we were familiar' (p. 176).

3 See Ayllon and Azrin, 1968, p. 217, for a list of visitors to the program and their programs. Noting the transportability of the token economy, they stated, 'The motivating environment was designed with the objective of generally applicability to different types of populations and different types of situations' (pp. 216–17). Their goal was to create a technology that not only could be transported across different physical settings, but could also be applied to a range of behavior problems. This transportability helped the spread of behavior modification generally.

4 See Ulmer, 1976, for a description of the Camarillo program; see Morisse, Batra, Hess, Silverman, and Corrigan, 1996, for a report of a more recently implemented program in Chicago.

4: Crime and Punishment: Contingency Management in the Prison System

1 Letter from B.F. Skinner to McGeorge Bundy of the Ford Foundation, 13 March 1970, Skinner Papers, HUG FP 60.10, Box 15, Folder: D-F Corr. 1965–71, HUA.

2 Although I focus my discussion on CASE, there were other important programs for juvenile delinquents initiated in this period. Achievement Place in Lawrence, Kansas, for example, was a community-based residential treatment program for pre-delinquent boys using a token economy (e.g., Phillips, 1968). For an overview of a number of these programs, including Achievement Place, see Burchard and Harig, 1976.

3 Israel Goldiamond to B.F. Skinner, 13 December 1962, Skinner Papers, HUG FP 60.10, Box 6, Folder: Misc. 1962, #1 of 2, HUA.

4 It is notable that the study cubicles were in fact large, customized boxes. As R. Buckminster Fuller wrote in his preface to Cohen and Filipczak's description of the project: 'Each student ... had a little paper house (an office) that had been manufactured out of corrugated paperboard, like a very large box for a piano or a big radio' (Fuller, 1971, p. xv).

5 The CASE programs built directly on Cohen's experience with the Experimental Freshman Year at SIU, but also on a programmed course that he and James

Filipczak had designed and implemented there (see Cohen, 1968, p. 21, note 1). In CASE II, students were taught using programmed instruction.

6 For the rest of the section, I refer exclusively to the CASE II project. CASE I was a pilot project, and all students in CASE I also participated in CASE II.

7 Interestingly, in their 1971 monograph, Cohen and Filipczak devote a chapter to cultural and interpersonal issues in the program and discuss some of the racial tensions that arose as both white southerners and black northerners asserted their identities, and attempted to prove their superiority (see pp. 83–5).

8 This practice was dropped at later stages of the program, when points could only be earned by measured performance and achievement.

9 In describing his approach, Cohen pointed out that although the 'American ideal' was that students should do their best at all times and that good grades would serve as their own reward, the student inmates at the NTS did not share this ideal. He noted that these students were interested in the immediate payoff of their behavior in terms of material and social reinforcers.

10 At the beginning of the program, each student was given three to five days of free room and board in the improved conditions of Jefferson Hall. After that time, they had to use points to pay rent on a private room or return to communal sleeping arrangements. They also had to use points in order to buy better food than the standard institutional fare.

11 Letter from B.F. Skinner to H.L. Cohen, 10 January 1968, Skinner Papers, HUG FP 60.20, Box 6, Folder: IBR 1961–72, HUA.

12 The superintendent of the NTS at the time of the CASE programs, Roy Gerard, became the warden of the Kennedy Youth Center. Gerard was supportive of Cohen's work at the NTS and oversaw similar programs at the Kennedy Youth Center. Gerard then became the assistant director of correctional programs in the Federal Bureau of Prisons and, in February of 1974, appeared at the Oversight Hearing on Behavior Modification Programs in the Federal Bureau of Prisons to testify in support of the controversial START program, which I will describe shortly.

13 One of the most popular reinforcers was the opportunity to get a personal photograph taken. Once a week, program staff would bring in a Polaroid camera, and almost every prisoner with enough credits would pose for at least one self-portrait (see Geller, Johnson, Hamlin, and Kennedy, 1977, p. 22).

14 See 'ACLU Scores Token Economy' (Trotter, 1974), and Geller's response to this article (Geller and Johnson, 1974).

15 APA press release, 15 February 1974, Stolz Papers, Box M1030, Folder: Stolz 1, AHAP.

16 Memorandum by Al Bandura to the Board of Directors, 22 March 1974, Stolz Papers, Box M1030, Folder: Stolz 1, AHAP.

17 Fred Strassburger to Leonard Krasner, 29 October 1975, Stolz Papers, Box M1030, Folder: Stolz 1, AHAP.

18 Minutes of the Commission on Behavior Modification meeting, 10–11 October 1974, p. 3, Stolz Papers, Box M1030, Folder Stolz 1, AHAP.

19 Memorandum by Stephanie Stolz to Serena Stier, 21 July 1975, Stolz Papers, Box M1030, Folder: Stolz 1, AHAP.

20 Hugh Lacey to Stephanie Stolz, 21 February 1978, Stolz Papers, Box M1030, Folder: Stolz 1, AHAP.

21 Stephanie Stolz to Hugh Lacey, 13 March 1978, Stolz Papers, Box M1030, Folder: Stolz 1, AHAP.

22 See the Federal Register, Vol. 43, pp. 53652–6, Rules and Regulations, Part 46, Protection of Human Subjects, Additional Protections Pertaining to Biomedical and Behavioral Research Involving Prisoners as Subjects.

23 Minutes of the Commission on Behavior Modification meeting, 13–14 February 1975, p. 6, Stolz Papers, Box M1030, Folder: Stolz 1, AHAP.

24 Notably, another group of activists who came out against behavior modification and other rehabilitative strategies in prisons argued that the whole nature of imprisonment should be questioned and the number and size of prisons greatly reduced (see McCrea, 1975).

5: How to *Really* Win Friends and Influence People: Skinnerian Principles in Self-Help

1 For Skinner, self-management became particularly important as he faced the physical and mental challenges of aging. For his advice on how to manage these challenges, including many personal examples, see Skinner and Vaughan, 1983.

2 This phrase is a play on the phrase 'giving psychology away,' used by APA president and cognitive psychologist George Miller in his 1969 presidential address, which was subsequently published in the *American Psychologist*. I describe pertinent aspects of Miller's article later in this chapter, but in short he discusses the advantages and dangers of using psychology to solve social problems.

3 According to Barbara Ehrenreich and Deirdre English in *For Her Own Good: Two Centuries of the Experts' Advice to Women*, the ascent of the scientific expert in America began in the Progressive Era (1890s–1920s). They further argue that scientism took hold as a substitute for religious fervor in this period, and that the laboratory became a 'temple of objectivity' from which science (they focus on medical science) could survey the world of man and nature and write prescriptions for moral and social, as well as physical, ills (Ehrenreich and English,

2005, p. 85). By the 1970s, the scientists certainly retained much of their expert status, and self-help, at least in the form of self-help groups, had become somewhat of a national obsession (see Katz, 1981).

4 Thomas Gieryn describes a scientific truth-spot as a physical place that in its very generality and reproducibility actually transcends place and achieves universal acceptance as a spot from which truth is generated. The scientist's laboratory, he argues, has become such a truth-spot (see Gieryn, 2002).

5 Israel Goldiamond to B.F. Skinner, 13 December 1962, Skinner Papers, HUG FP 60.10, Box 6, Folder: #1 of 2 Misc. 1962, HUA.

6 Norma Fullgrabe to C.B. Ferster, 29 December 1965, Ferster Papers, Box: Ferster Depot, Folder: Diet control, AHAP.

7 C.B. Ferster, 'The control of eating,' unpublished manuscript, Ferster Papers, Box: Ferster Depot, Folder: Diet control, AHAP.

8 Ferster, 'The control of eating,' p. 7.

9 Ferster, 'The control of eating,' p. 13.

10 A 1977 edited volume entitled *Behavioral Treatments of Obesity* includes sixteen reprinted articles published between 1962 and 1976 on self-control techniques alone (see Foreyt, 1977). In fact, if Ferster, Nurnberger, and Levitt's classic article is excluded, the remaining fifteen articles were all published between 1967 and 1976.

11 By 1990, it was in its sixth edition; the twentieth anniversary revision went through two printings.

12 However, the cultural influence of operant psychology as self-help should not be underestimated. As recently as 2008, journalist Amy Sutherland published a self-help book entitled *What Shamu Taught Me about Life, Love, and Marriage*, based on her real-life application of the operant principles successfully used in animal training (Sutherland, 2008). A *New York Times* on-line feature piece based on the book, *What Shamu Taught Me about a Happy Marriage*, was the most viewed and e-mailed article of 2006.

6: Living the Dream: Walden Two and the Laboratory of Life

1 B.F. Skinner to Lillian MacDonald, 21 March 1956, Skinner Papers, HUG FP 60.52, Walden Two correspondence, 1946–74, HUA. See also Bjork, 1993, pp. 146–7.

2 As his biographer Daniel Bjork has noted, Skinner was not prone to praising others' books, but evidently he was quite taken with E.F. Schumacher's now-classic *Small Is Beautiful* (Bjork, 1993, p. 259). Smith (1992) has written, 'Often lost in the controversy generated by *Walden Two* is the recognition that the Walden Two community itself embodied many practices that would

qualify as appropriate technology by the standards of contemporary critics of technology. It was a small community characterized by harmony with the natural environment, modest use of resources, and planned abstinence from consumer consumption' (p. 222).

3 However, in small corners of the community, Skinner's ghost lives on. When the author visited several years ago, a stylized, computer-generated image of Skinner appeared as a poster on a living-room wall at Harmony, one of the courtyard residences at Twin Oaks. Harmony was named after the Owenite community, New Harmony, formed in Indiana in 1825 by Robert Owen. In the hammock-weaving room, head-set connections hang from the ceiling at every work-station so that workers can listen to music (creating a reinforcing environment) without disturbing others – a suggestion adopted directly from Skinner's novel and practiced by him in his own study. At the time of writing, a link to a *Walden Two* fan site (http://www.twinoaks.org/clubs/walden-two/index.html) could be found at the home page for Twin Oaks (http://www.twinoaks.org/).

4 Although I focus on Twin Oaks and Los Horcones, there were a number of communities established around the same time by academic behaviorists, such as Walden Three, Lake Village, and Sunflower House. For descriptions of these communities, see Kuhlmann, 2005, pp. 51–77. For an account of the early days of Walden Three as told by a visitor to the community, see Bouvard, 1975, pp. 183–7. For a short article on Lake Village, see Altus, 1998. As Twin Oaks grew and became more established, it spawned a second wave of Walden Two–type communities that numbered more than two dozen (Kuhlmann, 2005, p. xii).

5 The Federation of Egalitarian Communities was established in 1976 and now includes seven member communities and several affiliates throughout the United States. The members are committed to non-violence, participatory government, non-discrimination, environmental responsibility, and healthy interpersonal relationships. In each community, all resources are held communally and products of members' labor are distributed equally or according to need.

6 Altus and Morris (2004), and others, have pointed out that Skinner's goal in writing *Walden Two* was not to provide a literal blueprint for how to set up a community, but rather to propose that the good life should be derived by using an experimental attitude towards developing social practices that work to enhance both individual and cultural survival. As Skinner himself put it in a 1979 letter to the members of East Wind, an offshoot of Twin Oaks: 'I am in fairly close touch with Los Horcones and of course appreciate the closeness with which they are following behavioristic principles, but *any way to work out the good life is okay with me*' (B.F. Skinner to 'my Friends at East Wind,' 13 December 1979, emphasis added, HUG FP 60.10, Box 27, Folder: E Corr 1974–9, 1 of 2, Skinner Papers, HUA). I use the term 'blueprint' here

because in their early attempts at setting up a community, Twin Oakers did look to *Walden Two* as a literal model for community, trying out several of the ideas Skinner presented in the form they appeared in the book.

7 C. Smith to B.F. Skinner, 24 May 1968, Skinner Papers, HUG FP 60.52, Walden Two correspondence, 1946–74, HUA.

8 Barry Burkan to B.F. Skinner, 28 June 1968, Skinner Papers, HUG FP 60.52, Walden Two correspondence, 1946–74, HUA.

9 S. Morgan to B.F. Skinner, 20 March 1966, Skinner Papers, HUG FP 60.52, Walden Two correspondence, 1946–74, HUA.

10 G. Griebe to B.F. Skinner, 19 June 1965, Skinner Papers, HUG FP 60.52, Walden Two correspondence, 1946–74, HUA.

11 J. Majewsky to B.F. Skinner, 21 March 1966, Skinner Papers, HUG FP 60.52, Walden Two correspondence, 1946–74, HUA.

12 B.F. Skinner to G. Griebe, 22 June 1965, Skinner Papers, HUG FP 60.52, Walden Two correspondence, 1946–74, HUA.

13 Experimental work on the effects of reinforcement on intrinsic motivation was not to appear until well after Skinner had devised his system (see, for example, Lepper, Greene, and Nisbett, 1973).

14 What has happened to the children raised at Twin Oaks? To my knowledge, there has been no published account systematically describing the fate of children raised in the community. However, Kinkade has remarked that most parents 'reach the end of their desire to be communal' by the time their children reach grade-school age. Of the three or four children who have stayed in the community until adolescence, Kinkade reported that they are 'pretty normal.' She wrote, 'They tend to seek each other out and remain friends for many years. What they say about Twin Oaks memories is that it is a wonderful place for children and they used to have lots of other kids to play with, and now they don't and sometimes are lonely' (Kinkade, personal communication, 17 November 2000). Interestingly, in her assessment, Kuhlmann (2005, pp. 102–6) notes that the communal child-rearing model envisioned in *Walden Two* did not work at Twin Oaks, despite a variety of efforts to implement it. In fact, Kuhlmann quotes Kat Kinkade's own granddaughter, Lee Ann Kinkade, as reporting that she found it emotionally difficult to deal with the high turnover in child-care workers during the first five years of her life: 'I got very used to losing people' (as cited in Kuhlmann, 2005, p. 106).

15 Kinkade offered the following assessment of Skinner's interest in Twin Oaks: 'Skinner was a kind, warm, self-centered man who disappointed me, mostly because he didn't turn out to be Frazier. He was interested in his own field, and the field of community building didn't interest him. He read my first book, was very congratulatory about it, and consented to write a

foreword for it. He came to Twin Oaks only once, as part of his arrangement to appear on the NOVA show. They filmed him here. He said polite things about us, but it was obvious that it was behaviorism he cared about, not community' (K. Kinkade, personal communication, 23 May 1999).

16 See, for example, B.F. Skinner to C.W. Moslander, 31 July 1974, Skinner Papers, HUG FP 60.20 Box 15, Twin Oaks correspondence, 1974–9, HUA.

17 Piper to B.F. Skinner, 26 March 1977, Skinner Papers, HUG FP 60.20 Box 15, Twin Oaks correspondence, 1974–9, HUA.

18 B.F. Skinner to C.W. Moslander, 31 July 1974, Skinner Papers, HUG FP 60.20 Box 15, Twin Oaks correspondence, 1974–9, HUA.

19 B.F. Skinner to Gerri, 7 November 1978, Skinner Papers, HUG FP 60.20 Box 15, Twin Oaks correspondence, 1974–9, HUA.

20 B.F. Skinner to David Ruth, 25 July 1977, Skinner Papers, HUG FP 60.20 Box 15, Twin Oaks correspondence, 1974–9, HUA.

21 David Ruth, 'On B.F. Skinner's First Visit to Twin Oaks, Turnover, and the Meaning of Life,' 1976, unpublished manuscript, Skinner Papers, HUG FP 60.20 Box 15, Twin Oaks correspondence, 1974–9, HUA. Skinner later requested that this information be omitted from the report, preferring his loan to remain anonymous. There is also indirect evidence that he later converted the loan to a donation, perhaps for the purposes of purchasing the television and recording equipment mentioned above.

22 B.F. Skinner to Gerri, 22 September 1978, Skinner Papers, HUG FP 60.20 Box 15, Twin Oaks correspondence, 1974–9, HUA.

23 B.F. Skinner to David Ruth, 21 January 1977, Skinner Papers, HUG FP 60.20 Box 15, Twin Oaks correspondence, 1974–9, HUA.

24 The Spanish word 'horcones' refers to the wood pillars used by the community to support the tile roofs of many of their buildings. More symbolically, the word is used by the community to connote the pillars of a new society.

25 Again, there has been no systematic, follow-up study of children raised and educated at Los Horcones. However, the first child in the community was Juan Robinson-Bustamente, the son of two of the founders, Juan Robinson and Mireya Bustamente. He is now twenty-nine years old and continues to live in the community with his wife, whom he met there. He is ardently committed to the community and to the application of the science of behavior. For further information, see Altus, 1999.

Conclusion: From Laboratory to Life

1 I have not systematically covered the history of applied behavior analysis and autism. Today, this is an extremely important stronghold of behavior-analytic

expertise. The Work of O. Ivar Lovaas was pioneering and particularly important in this area. Readers are referred to his monograph *The Autistic Child* (1977).

2 For a review of this work, see Lehman and Geller, 2004. Interestingly, these authors note that despite the demonstrated power of behavioral technology in engineering environmental preservation, the field has nonetheless been limited in terms of its widespread impact. They cite several reasons for this and conclude by giving a number of practical suggestions for how to increase this impact.

3 See Bailey and Gillespy, 2005, for a history of Marian and Keller Breland's application of operant psychology to commercial animal training; see Pryor, 1999, for a widely used dog training manual with operant roots.

4 Interestingly, one could argue that applied behavior analysis has ultimately experienced its most marked success with the very same subjects who were originally placed inside the human Skinner box: autistic and developmentally delayed children, young school kids, and psychiatric patients.

5 There are obviously other psychological approaches that have claimed the status of technologies, or that have been referred to as psychotechnologies, such as testing, other non-behavioral forms of therapy, psychological practices applied to business and industry, etc. My intent is not to make a priority claim for Skinner's use of the term 'technology' or to suggest that his system was unique in its technological aspect. I am suggesting, however, that in the American context, Skinner's approach was perhaps one of the most explicitly and thoroughly technological in its orientation and terminology, that it benefitted significantly from its resonance with the American technological imperative, and, as Smith (1992) has ably discussed, has also seen its fortunes tied to the rise *and* fall of technological enthusiasm in the United States. Further, I propose that it is appropriate to historically and conceptually situate Skinner's technology of behavior among the technologies of the self that have been defined by historians and philosophers more broadly as strategies which 'permit individuals to effect by their own means or with the help of others a certain number of operations on their own bodies and souls, thoughts, conduct, and way of being, so as to transform themselves' (Foucault, 1988, p. 18).

References

Ader, R., and Tatum, R. (1961). Free-operant avoidance conditioning in human subjects. *Journal of the Experimental Analysis of Behavior, 4*, 275–6.

Adler, J. (2006, March 27). Freud in our midst. *Newsweek.* Retrieved 29 August 2007 from: http://www.msnbc.msn.com/id/11904222/site/newsweek/

Agnew's blast at behaviorism. (1972, January). *Psychology Today, 4*, 84, 87.

Alberti, R.E., and Emmons, M.L. (1974). *Your perfect right: A guide to assertive behavior.* San Luis Obispo, CA: IMPACT.

Alexander, D. (2004, July 9). Interview with Duane Alexander, M.D. Oral history of the Belmont Report and the National Commission for the Protection of Human Subjects of Biomedical and Behavioral Research, Belmont Oral History Project. Retrieved 13 July 2005 from: http://www.hhs.gov/ohrp/docs/InterviewAlexander.doc

Allen, K.E., Hart, B., Buell, J.S., Harris, F.R., and Wolf, M.M. (1964). Effects of social reinforcement on isolate behavior of a nursery school child. *Child Development, 35*, 511–18.

Altus, D.E. (1998, Spring). Roger Ulrich and Lake Village Community: The 'experiment of life.' *Communities: A Journal of Cooperative Living, 98*, 52–4.

– (1999, Summer). Growing up at Los Horcones. *Communities: A Journal of Cooperative Living, 103*, 53–7.

Altus, D.E., Kuhlmann, H., and Welsh, T. (1999, Summer). Walden Two communities: Where are they now? *Communities: A Journal of Cooperative Living, 103*, 27–8.

Altus, D.E., and Morris, E.K. (2004). B.F. Skinner's utopian vision: Behind and beyond *Walden Two. Contemporary Justice Review, 7*, 267–86.

Atthowe, J.M., and Krasner, L. (1968). Preliminary report on the application of contingent reinforcement procedures (token economy) on a 'chronic' psychiatric ward. *Journal of Abnormal Psychology, 73*, 37–43.

Ayllon, T. (2005, April 8). Interview with the author, Atlanta, GA.

Ayllon, T., and Azrin, N.H. (1965). The measurement and reinforcement of behavior of psychotics. *Journal of the Experimental Analysis of Behavior, 8*, 357–83.

– (1968). *The token economy: A motivational system for therapy and rehabilitation.* New York: Appleton-Century-Crofts.

Ayllon, T., and Haughton, E. (1962). Control of the behavior of schizophrenic patients by food. *Journal of the Experimental Analysis of Behavior, 5*, 343–52.

Ayllon, T., and Michael, J. (1959). The psychiatric nurse as a behavioral engineer. *Journal of the Experimental Analysis of Behavior, 2*, 323–34.

Azrin, N., and Lindsley, O. (1956). The reinforcement of cooperation between children. *Journal of Abnormal and Social Psychology, 52*, 100–2.

Baby box. (1947, July 19). *New Yorker,* 19–20.

Bailey, R.E., and Gillespy, J.A. (2005). Operant psychology goes to the fair: Marian and Keller Breland in the popular press. *Behavior Analyst, 28*, 143–59.

Barash, D.P. (2005, April 1). B.F. Skinner, revisited. *Chronicle of Higher Education,* B10–11.

Baron, A., and Perone, M. (1982). The place of the human subject in the operant laboratory. *Behavior Analyst, 5*, 143–58.

Barton, W.E., and Sanborn, C.J. (1977). *An assessment of the Community Mental Health Movement.* Lexington, MA: Lexington Books.

Behavior Modification Programs, Federal Bureau of Prisons: Hearing before the Subcommittee on Courts, Civil Liberties, and the Administration of Justice of the Committee on the Judiciary House of Representatives, 93 Cong. (1974, February 27).

Bell, J.N. (1961, October). Will robots teach your children? *Popular mechanics,* 153–7, 246.

Benjamin, L.T. (1988). A history of teaching machines. *American Psychologist, 43,* 703–12.

Benjamin, L.T., and Nielsen-Gammon, E. (1999). B.F. Skinner and psychotechnology: The case of the heir conditioner. *Review of General Psychology, 3,* 155–67.

Bijou, S.W. (1955). A systematic approach to the experimental analysis of young children. *Child Development, 26,* 161–8.

– (1957). Methodology for an experimental analysis of child behaviors. *Psychological Reports, 3,* 243–50.

– (1959). A child study laboratory on wheels. *Child Development, 29,* 425–7.

– (2001). Child behavior therapy: Early history. In W.J. O'Donohue, D.A. Henderson, S.C. Hayes, J.E. Fisher, and L.J. Hayes (Eds.), *A history of the behavioral therapies: Founders' personal histories* (pp. 105–24). Reno, NV: Context Press.

Biklen, D.P. (1976). Behavior modification in a state mental hospital: A participant-observer's critique. *American Journal of Orthopsychiatry, 46,* 53–61.

Birnbrauer, J.S. (1978). Better living through behaviorism? *Journal of Applied Behavior Analysis, 11,* 176–7.

Birnbrauer, J.S., and Lawler, J. (1964). Token reinforcement for learning. *Mental Retardation, 2,* 275–9.

Bjork, D.W. (1993). *B.F. Skinner: A life.* New York: Basicbooks.

– (1996). B.F. Skinner and the American tradition: The scientist as social inventor. In L.D. Smith and W.R. Woodward (Eds.), *B.F. Skinner and behaviorism in American culture* (pp. 128–50). Bethlehem, PA: Lehigh University Press.

Blakeslee, S. (1975, April 29). M.I.T. researcher studies 'visible scientists' and impact they have on public issues. *New York Times,* 21.

Boehm, G.A. (1960, October). Can people be taught like pigeons? *Fortune, 176,* 179, 259–60, 265–6.

Boroff, D. (1963, February). Education comes of age. *Parents' Magazine, 38,* 74, 116, 118, 120.

Bouvard, M. (1975). *The intentional community movement: Building a new moral world.* Port Washington, NY: Kennikat Press.

Box-bred babies. (1963, February 15). *Time,* 72.

Box-reared babies: Skinner baby-box (1954, February 22). *Time,* 66.

Boxes for babies. (1947, November 3). *Life,* 73–4.

Budd, W.C. (1973). *Behavior modification: The scientific way to self-control.* Roslyn Heights, NY: Libra Publishers.

Buhle, M.J. (1998). *Feminism and its discontents: A century of struggle with psychoanalysis.* Cambridge, MA: Harvard University Press.

Burchard, J.D., and Harig, P.T. (1976). Behavior modification and juvenile delinquency. In H. Leitenberg (Ed.), *Handbook of behavior modification and behavior therapy* (pp. 405–52). Englewood Cliffs, NJ: Prentice-Hall.

Burgess, A. (1972, February 17). Clockwork marmalade. *Listener, 87,* 197–9.

Burnham, J.C. (1987). *How superstition won and science lost: Popularizing science and health in the United States.* New Brunswick, NJ: Rutgers University Press.

Buskist, W.F., and Miller, H.L. (1982). The study of human operant behavior, 1958–1981: A topical bibliography. *Psychological Record, 32,* 249–68.

Campbell, R.F. (1967, January 14). Tomorrow's teacher. *Saturday Review, 60,* 62–4, 73.

Capshew, J.H. (1992). Psychologists on site: A reconnaissance of the historiography of the laboratory. *American Psychologist, 47,* 132–42.

– (1996). Engineering behavior: Project Pigeon, World War II, and the conditioning of B.F. Skinner. In L.D. Smith and W.R. Woodward (Eds.), *B.F. Skinner and behaviorism in American culture* (pp. 128–50). Bethlehem, PA: Lehigh University Press.

– (1999). *Psychologists on the march: Science, practice, and professional identity in America, 1929–1969.* Cambridge: Cambridge University Press.

Carlson, C.G., Hersen, M., and Eisler, R.M. (1972). Token economy programs in the treatment of hospitalized adult psychiatric patients: Current status and recent trends. *Journal of Nervous and Mental Disease, 155,* 192–204.

Catania, A.C. (2002). The watershed years of 1958–1962 in the Harvard Pigeon Lab. *Journal of the Experimental Analysis of Behavior, 77,* 327–45.

Chance, P. (1999, Summer). Science of behavior, sí! *Communities: A Journal of Cooperative Living, 103,* 29–34.

Chomsky, N. (1959). [Review of the book *Verbal behaviour.*] *Language, 35,* 26–58.

Clements, C.B., and McKee, J.M. (1968). Programmed instruction for institutionalized offenders: Contingency management and performance contracts. *Psychological Reports, 22,* 957–64.

Cohen, H.L. (1968). Educational therapy: The design of learning environments. In J.M. Schlien (Ed.), *Research in psychotherapy, Vol. 3* (pp. 21–53). Washington, DC: American Psychological Association.

– (1972). Programming alternatives to punishment: The design of competence through consequences. In S. Bijou and E. Ribes-Inesta (Eds.), *Behavior modification: Issues and extensions* (pp. 63–84). Oxford: Academic Press.

– (1976). BPLAY: A community support system, Phase one. In E. Ribes-Inesta and A. Bandura (Eds.), *Analysis of delinquency and aggression* (pp. 147–69). Oxford: Erlbaum.

Cohen, H. L., and Filipczak, J. (1971). *A new learning environment: A case for learning.* Boston: Authors Cooperative.

Coleman, S.R. (1984). Background and change in B.F. Skinner's metatheory from 1930 to 1938. *Journal of Mind and Behavior, 5,* 471–500.

– (1991). From critic to theorist: Themes in Skinner's development from 1928 to 1938. *Journal of Mind and Behavior, 12,* 509–34.

Comunidad Los Horcones. (1982). Pilot Walden Two experiments: Beginnings of a planned society. *Behaviorists for Social Action Journal, 3,* 25–9.

– (1989). Walden Two and social change: The application of behavior analysis to cultural design. *Behavior Analysis and Social Action, 7,* 35–41.

– (1999a, June 10). *Brief introduction to Los Horcones Community.* Retrieved 29 August 2007 from: http://www.loshorcones.org.mx/introduction.html

– (1999b, December 10). *Communitarian family.* Retrieved 29 August 2007 from: http://www.loshorcones.org.mx/family.html

– (1999c, April 5). *Labor area.* Retrieved 29 August 2007 from: http://www.loshorcones.org.mx/labor.html

– (1999d, December 2). *Personocracy: A government of the people, for the people, and by the people as individual persons.* Retrieved 29 August 2007 from: http://www.loshorcones.org.mx/government.html

– (1999e, May). Western culture influences in behaviour analysis seen from a Walden Two. Paper presented at the 25th Annual Convention of the Association for Behavior Analysis, Chicago, IL.

Coon, D.J. (1992). Testing the limits of sense and science: American experimental psychologists combat spiritualism, 1880–1920. *American Psychologist, 47*, 143–51.

The critics speak – teaching machines: What's ahead? (1967, September). *Today's Health*, 56–7.

Crowe, B. (1969). The tragedy of the commons revisited. *Science, 166*, 1103–7.

Cuban, L. (1986). *Teachers and machines: The classroom use of technology since 1920.* New York: Teachers' College Press.

Curti, M. (1980). *Human nature in American thought: A history.* Madison: University of Wisconsin Press.

Cushman, P. (1995). *Constructing the self, constructing America: A cultural history of psychotherapy.* Reading, MA: Addison-Wesley.

Danziger, K. (1990). *Constructing the subject: Historical origins of psychological research.* Cambridge: Cambridge University Press.

– (1997). *Naming the mind: How psychology found its language.* London: Sage.

Day, W.F. (1983). On the difference between radical and methodological behaviorism. *Behaviorism, 11*, 89–102.

Day, W.F., and Moore, J. (1995). On certain relations between contemporary philosophy and radical behaviorism. In J.T. Todd and E.K. Morris (Eds.), *Modern perspectives on B.F. Skinner and contemporary behaviorism* (pp. 75–84). Westport, CT: Greenwood Press.

DeBell, C.S., and Harless, D.K. (1992). B.F. Skinner: Myth and misperception. *Teaching of Psychology, 19*, 68–73.

Delprato, D.J., and Midgley, B.D. (1992). Some fundamentals of Skinner's behaviorism. *American Psychologist, 47*, 1507–20.

Dewsbury, D. (2003). Conflicting approaches: Operant psychology arrives at a primate laboratory. *Behavior Analyst, 26*, 253–65.

– (2006). *Monkey farm: A history of the Yerkes Laboratories of Primate Biology at Orange Park, Florida, 1930–1965.* Lewisburg, PA: Bucknell University Press.

Dickerson, F.B., Tenhula, W.N., and Green-Paden, L.D. (2005). The token economy for schizophrenia: Review of the literature and recommendations for future research. *Schizophrenia Research, 75*, 405–16.

Dickinson, B. (1971, November). [Letter to the editor.] *Psychology Today, 4*, 6, 8, 104.

Dinsmoor, J.A. (1982). Charles B. Ferster (1922–1981). *American Psychologist, 37*, 235.

– (1992). Setting the record straight: The social views of B.F. Skinner. *American Psychologist, 47*, 1454–63.

Ehrenreich, B., and English, D. (2005). *For her own good: Two centuries of the experts' advice to women.* Revised edition. New York: Random House.

Electronic instruction: Blessing or curse? (1966, October 5). *Christian Century*, 1201.

Elms, A.C. (1981). Skinner's dark year and Walden Two. *American Psychologist, 36*, 470–9.

182   References

Epting, L.K. (2008). Quiet influences, big consequences: An interview with Carol Pilgrim. *Teaching of Psychology, 35*, 51–8.

Falk, J.L. (1958). The grooming behavior of the chimpanzee as a reinforcer. *Journal of the Experimental Analysis of Behavior, 1*, 83–5.

Ferster, C.B. (1953). The use of the free operant in the analysis of behavior. *Psychological Bulletin, 50*, 263–74.

– (1957). Concurrent schedules of reinforcement in the chimpanzee. *Science, 125*, 1090–1.

– (1958). Intermittent reinforcement of a complex response in a chimpanzee. *Journal of the Experimental Analysis of Behavior, 1*, 163–5.

– (1961). Positive reinforcement and behavioral deficits of autistic children. *Child Development, 32*, 437–56.

– (2002/1970). Schedules of reinforcement with Skinner. *Journal of the Experimental Analysis of Behavior, 77*, 303–11.

Ferster, C.B., and DeMyer, M.K. (1961). The development of performances in autistic children in an automatically controlled environment. *Journal of Chronic Diseases, 13*, 312–45.

– (1962). A method for the experimental analysis of the behavior of autistic children. *American Journal of Orthopsychiatry, 3*, 89–98.

Ferster, C.B., Nurnberger, J.I., and Levitt, E.E. (1977). The control of eating. In J.P. Foreyt (Ed.), *Behavioral treatments of obesity* (pp. 309–26). Oxford: Pergamon Press. (Reprinted from *Journal of Mathetics, 1*, 87–109, 1962.)

Ferster, C.B., and Skinner, B.F. (1957). *Schedules of reinforcement.* New York: Appleton-Century-Crofts.

Foreyt, J.P. (Ed.). (1977). *Behavioral treatments of obesity.* Oxford: Pergamon Press.

Foucault, M. (1988). Technologies of the self. In L.H. Martin, H. Gutman, and P.H. Hutton (Eds.), *Technologies of the self: A seminar with Michel Foucault* (pp. 16–49). London: Tavistock Publications.

Fox, D.R. (1985). Psychology, ideology, utopia, and the commons. *American Psychologist, 40*, 48–58.

Freedom and funding: Skinner support queried. (1971, December 25). *Science News*, 420–1.

Fuller, R.B. (1971). Foreword. In H.L. Cohen and J. Filipczak, *A new learning environment* (pp. xi-xvi). San Francisco: Jossey-Bass.

Fuller, R.C. (1982). Carl Rogers, religion, and the role of psychology in American culture. *Journal of Humanistic Psychology, 22*, 21–32.

Fuller, P.R. (1949). Operant conditioning of a vegetative human organism. *American Journal of Psychology, 62*, 587–90.

Gabbard, G., and Gabbard, K. (1999). *Psychiatry and the cinema.* 2nd ed. Washington, DC: American Psychological Association.

Geller, E.S. (2001). Behavior-based safety in industry: Realizing the large-scale potential of psychology to promote human welfare. *Applied and Preventive Psychology, 10*, 87–105.

– (2005). Behavior-based safety and occupational risk management. *Behavior Modification, 29*, 539–61.

– (2005, December 2). Interview with the author, Blacksburg, VA.

Geller, E.S., and Johnson, D.F. (1974, November). [Letter to the editor.] *APA Monitor, 5*, 5.

Geller, E.S., Johnson, D.F., Hamlin, P.H., and Kennedy, T.D. (1977). Behavior modification in a prison: Issues, problems, and compromises. *Criminal Justice and Behavior, 4*, 11–43.

Gieryn, T. (2002). Three truth spots. *Journal of the History of the Behavioral Sciences, 38*, 113–32.

Gilmore, K. (1961, February). Teaching machines – blessing or curse? *Science Digest*, 76–80.

Glynn, S.M. (1990). Token economy approaches for psychiatric patients: Progress and pitfalls over 25 years. *Behavior Modification, 14*, 383–407.

Goldiamond, I. (1965). Self-control procedures in personal behavior problems. *Psychological Reports, 17*, 851–68.

– (1973). Self-control procedures in personal behavior problems. In M.R. Goldfried and M. Merbaum (Eds.), *Behavior change through self-control* (pp. 268–86). New York: Holt, Rinehart and Winston, Inc.

Golinski, J. (2005). *Making natural knowledge: Constructivism and the history of science*. Chicago: University of Chicago Press.

Goodall, K. (1972, November). Shapers at work. *Psychology Today, 6*, 53–63, 132–8.

Goodell, R. (1977). *The visible scientists*. Boston: Little, Brown and Company.

Greenwood, J.D. (1999). Understanding the 'cognitive revolution' in psychology. *Journal of the History of the Behavioral Sciences, 35*, 1–22.

Gripp, R.F., and Magaro, P.A. (1971). A token economy program evaluated with untreated control ward comparisons. *Behaviour Research and Therapy, 9*, 137–49.

Hacking, I. (1995). Looping effects of human kinds. In D. Sperber, D. Premack, and A.J. Premack (Eds.), *Causal cognition: A multidisciplinary debate* (pp. 351–94). New York: Oxford University Press.

Haggbloom, S.J., Warnick, R., Warnick, J.E., Jones, V.K., Yarbrough, G.L., et al. (2002). The 100 most eminent psychologists of the 20th century. *Review of General Psychology, 6*, 139–52.

Hale, N.G. (1995). The 'golden-age' of popularization, 1945–1965. In N.G. Hale, *The rise and crisis of psychoanalysis in the United States* (pp. 276–99). New York: Oxford University Press.

Hall, E. (1972, November). My hat still fits. *Psychology Today, 6*, 68.

Hall, J.N. (1973). Ward behaviour modification projects in Great Britain. *Bulletin of the British Psychological Society, 26,* 199–201.

Hall, J.N., and Baker, R. (1973). Token economy systems: Breakdown and control. *Behavior Research and Therapy, 11,* 253–63.

Harris, F.R., Johnston, M.K., Kelley, C.S., and Wolf, M.M. (1964). Effects of positive social reinforcement on regressed crawling of a nursery school child. *Journal of Educational Psychology, 55,* 35–41.

Heated, air-conditioned 'baby box' aids mothers. (1948, March 17). *Indianapolis News.*

Herman, E. (1992). Being and doing: Humanistic psychology and the spirit of the 1960s. In B.L. Tischler (Ed.), *Sights on the sixties.* New Brunswick, NJ: Rutgers University Press.

– (1995). *The romance of American psychology: Political culture in the age of experts.* Berkeley and Los Angeles: University of California Press.

Hilts, P.J. (1973a, April 29). The controllers. *Washington Post Potomac,* 18.

– (1973b, April 29). Mastering yourself. *Washington Post Potomac,* 21, 38, 41.

– (1974). *Behavior mod.* New York: Harper's Magazine Press.

Hobbs, S., Cornwell, D., and Chiesa, M. (2000). Telling tales about behavior analysis: Textbooks, scholarship and rumor. In J.C. Leslies and D. Blackman (Eds.), *Experimental and applied analysis of human behavior* (pp. 251–70). Reno, NV: Context Press.

Holland, J. (1976). Ethical considerations in behavior modification. *Journal of Humanistic Psychology, 16,* 71–8.

Holland, J.G. (1978). Behaviorism: Part of the problem or part of the solution? *Journal of Applied Behavior Analysis, 11,* 163–74.

Holland, J.S. (1978). A critique of the use of behavior modification in prisons. In S.B. Stolz and Associates, *Ethical issues in behavior modification* (pp. 73–89). San Francisco: Jossey-Bass.

Horgan, J. (1996, December). Why Freud isn't dead. *Scientific American, 275(4),* 106–11.

How a tech professor raises his youngsters in a 'baby box.' (1954, March 7). *Boston Sunday Globe.*

Ice cream for the right answers. (1968, August 1). *Forbes,* 46.

Individual rights and the federal role in behavior modification: A study. (1974, November). Prepared by the Staff of the Subcommittee on Constitutional Rights of the Committee on the Judiciary, United States Senate, Ninety-third Congress, Second Session. Washington, DC: U.S. Government Printing Office.

Is freedom obsolete. (1971, September 11). *New York Times,* 26.

Jastrow, J. (1889). The problems of 'psychic research.' *Harper's New Monthly Magazine, 79,* 76–82.

– (1928). *Keeping mentally fit.* New York: Garden City Publishing Co.

Jordan, E.A. (1996). Freedom and the control of children: The Skinners' approach to parenting. In L.D. Smith and W.R. Woodward (Eds.), *B.F. Skinner and behaviorism in American culture* (pp. 199–213). Bethlehem, PA: Lehigh University Press.

Kale, R.J., Zlutnick, S., and Hopkins, B.L. (1968). Patient contributions to a therapeutic environment. *Michigan Mental Health Research Bulletin, 2,* 33–8.

Kanfer, F.H. (1965). Issues and ethics in behavior manipulation. *Psychological Reports, 16,* 187–96.

Kanter, R.M. (1972). *Commitment and community: Communes and utopias in sociological perspective.* Cambridge, MA: Harvard University Press.

Kantor, J.R. (1968). Behaviorism in the history of psychology. *Psychological Record, 18,* 151–66.

Katz, A.H. (1981). Self-help and mutual aid: An emerging social movement? *Annual Review of Sociology, 7,* 129–55.

Kazdin, A.E. (1974). Self-monitoring and behavior change. In M.J. Mahoney and C.E. Thoresen (Eds.), *Self-control: Power to the person* (pp. 218–46). Monterey, CA: Brooks/Cole Publishing Company.

– (1977). *The token economy: A review and evaluation.* New York: Plenum Press.

– (1978). *History of behavior modification: Experimental foundations of contemporary research.* Baltimore: University Park Press.

– (1982). History of behavior modification. In A.S. Bellack, M.S. Hersen, and A.E. Kazdin (Eds.), *International handbook of behavior modification and therapy* (pp. 3–32). New York: Plenum Press.

Kazdin, A.E., and Bootzin, R. (1972). The token economy: An evaluative review. *Journal of Applied Behavior Analysis, 5,* 343–72.

Kelleher, R.T. (1957). A multiple schedule of conditioned reinforcement with chimpanzees. *Psychological Reports, 3,* 485–91.

Kinkade, K. (1973). *A Walden Two experiment.* New York: Quill.

– (1994). *Is it utopia yet?* Louisa, VA: Twin Oaks Publishing.

– (1999, Summer). But can he design community? *Communities: A Journal of Cooperative Living, 103,* 49–52.

Knapp, T.J. (1996). The verbal legacy of B.F. Skinner: An essay on the secondary literature. In L.D. Smith and W.R. Woodward (Eds.), *B.F. Skinner and behaviorism in American culture* (pp. 273–93). Bethlehem, PA: Lehigh University Press.

Komar, I. (1983). *Living the dream: A documentary study of the Twin Oaks community.* Norwood, PA: Norwood Editions.

Korn, J.H., Davis, R., and Davis, S.F. (1991). Historians' and chairpersons' judgments of eminence among psychologists. *American Psychologist, 46,* 789–92.

Krantz, D.L. (1972). Schools and systems: The mutual isolation of operant and non-operant psychology as a case study. *Journal of the History of the Behavioral Sciences, 8,* 86–102.

Krasner, L. (1962). Behavior control and social responsibility. *American Psychologist, 17*, 199–204.

– (1977). An interview with Sidney W. Bijou. In B.C. Etzel, J.M. LeBlanc, and D.M. Baer (Eds.), *New developments in behavioral research: Theory, method, and application* (pp. 587–99). Hillsdale, NJ: Erlbaum.

– (1990). History of behavior modification. In A.S. Bellack, M.S. Hersen, and A.E. Kazdin (Eds.), *International handbook of behavior modification and therapy*, 2nd ed. (pp. 3–25). New York: Plenum Press.

Krasner, L., and Krasner, M. (1973). Token economies and other planned environments. In C.E. Thoresen (Ed.), *Behavior modification in education* (pp. 351–81). Chicago: University of Chicago Press.

Kreig, M.B. (1961, February). What about teaching machines? *Parents' Magazine*, 44–5, 76, 78, 80.

Kroker, K. (2003). The progress of introspection in America, 1896–1938. *Studies in History and Philosophy of Biological and Biomedical Sciences, 34*, 77–108.

Kuhlmann, H. (1999a, Summer). Walden Two communities: What were they all about? *Communities: A Journal of Cooperative Living, 103*, 35–41.

– (1999b, Summer). 'Who's the meta tonight?': Communal child rearing at Twin Oaks. *Communities: A Journal of Cooperative Living, 103*, 45–8.

– (2005). *Living Walden Two: B.F. Skinner's behaviorist utopia and experimental communities.* Urbana and Chicago: University of Illinois Press.

Kumar, K. (1991). *Utopianism.* Minneapolis: University of Minnesota Press.

La Follette, M.G. (1990). *Making science our own: Public images of science, 1910–1955.* Chicago and London: University of Chicago Press.

Lamal, P.A. (1989). The impact of behaviorism on our culture: Some evidence and conjectures. *Psychological Record, 39*, 529–35.

Laties, V.G. (2003). Behavior analysis and the growth of behavioral pharmacology. *Behavior Analyst, 26*, 235–52.

Laties, V.G., and Mace, F.C. (1993). Taking stock: The first 25 years of the *Journal of Applied Behavior Analysis. Journal of Applied Behavior Analysis, 26*, 513–25.

Latour, B. (1987). *Science in action: How to follow scientists and engineers through society.* Cambridge, MA: Harvard University Press.

Latour, B., and Woolgar, S. (1986). *Laboratory life: The construction of scientific facts.* 2nd ed. Princeton, NJ: Princeton University Press.

Lattal, K. (2004). Steps and pips in the history of the cumulative recorder. *Journal of the Experimental Analysis of Behavior, 82*, 329–55.

Leahey, T.H. (1992). The mythical revolutions of American psychology. *American Psychologist, 47*, 308–18.

– (2001). *A history of modern psychology.* Englewood Cliffs, NJ: Prentice-Hall.

Leary, D.E. (1987). Telling likely stories: The rhetoric of the New Psychology, 1880–1920. *Journal of the History of the Behavioral Sciences, 23*, 315–31.

Lee, J. (1983, October 10). Still walking faster and longer. *Time*, 42, 43.

Lehman, P.K., and Geller, E.S. (2004). Behavior analysis and environmental protection: Accomplishments and potential for more. *Journal of Social Issues, 13*, 13–32.

Lehmann-Haupt, C. (1971, September 22). Skinner's design for living [Review of the book *Beyond freedom and dignity*]. *New York Times*, 45.

Lemov, R. (2005). *World as laboratory: Experiments with mice, mazes, and men.* New York: Hill and Wang.

Lent, J.R. (1968, June). Mimosa Cottage: Experiment in hope. *Psychology Today, 2*, 51–8.

Lepper, M.R., Greene, D., and Nisbett, R.E. (1973). Undermining childrens' intrinsic interest with extrinsic reward: A test of the 'overjustification' hypothesis. *Journal of Personality and Social Psychology, 28*, 129–37.

Levison, R. (1974, June). [Letter to the editor.] *APA Monitor, 5*, 3.

Lieber, L. (1962, August 12). Bringing up baby in a magic box! *This Week Magazine, 7*, 8.

Lindsley, O.R. (1956). Operant conditioning methods applied to research in chronic schizophrenia. *Psychiatric Research Reports, 5*, 118–39.

– (1962). Operant conditioning techniques in the measurement of psychopharmacologic response. In J.H. Nodine and J.H. Moyer (Eds.), *Psychosomatic medicine: The first Hahnemann symposium* (pp. 373–83). Philadelphia: Lea and Febiger.

– (2001). Studies in behavior therapy and Behavior Research Laboratory: June 1953–1965. In W.J. O'Donohue, D.A. Henderson, S.C. Hayes, J.E. Fisher, and L.J. Hayes (Eds.), *A history of the behavioral therapies: Founders' personal histories* (pp. 125–53). Reno, NV: Context Press.

– (2002). Our Harvard pigeon, rat, dog, and human lab. *Journal of the Experimental Analysis of Behavior, 77*, 385–7.

– (2004, May 28). Interview with the author, Boston, MA.

Long, E.R., Hammack, J.T., May, F., and Campbell, B.J. (1958). Intermittent reinforcement of operant behavior in children. *Journal of the Experimental Analysis of Behavior, 1*, 315–39.

Lovaas, O.I. (1977). *The autistic child: Language development through behaviour modification.* New York: Irvington Publishers, Inc.

Mabry, J.H. (1996). Remembering: An anecdotal account of my graduate student years. *Behavior and Social Issues, 6(2)*, 109–25.

Mahoney, M.J., and Thoresen, C.E. (Eds.). (1974). *Self-control: Power to the person.* Monterey, CA: Brooks/Cole Publishing Company.

Malagodi, E.F. (1986). On radicalizing behaviorism: A call for cultural analysis. *Behavior Analyst, 9*, 1–17.

Mandler, G. (2007). *A history of modern experimental psychology: From James and Wundt to cognitive science.* Cambridge, MA: MIT Press.

Marling, K.A. (1994). *As seen on TV: The visual culture of everyday life in the 1950s.* Cambridge, MA: Harvard University Press.

Martin, G., and Pear, J. (1978). *Behavior modification: What it is and how to do it.* Englewood Cliffs, NJ: Prentice-Hall.

Martin, M. (1972). Behavior modification in the mental hospital: Assumptions and criticisms. *Hospital and Community Psychiatry, 23,* 287–9.

Martin, R., and Barresi, J. (2006). *The rise and fall of soul and self: An intellectual history of personal identity.* New York: Columbia University Press.

McCarry, C. (1971, November). He envisions a happier age. *McCall's,* 35.

McCrea, R. (1975, July 7). Modification and its discontents: The National Conference on Behavioral Issues in Closed Institutions. *APF Reporter.* Retrieved on 12 July 2005 from: http://www.aliciapatterson.org/APF001975/McCrea/McCrea02/McCrea02.html#3

McFarling, U.L. (2000, May 15). Freud slips as icon of science. *Los Angeles Times,* A1, A8.

McKee, J.M., and Clements, C.B. (1971). A behavioral approach to learning: The Draper model. In H.C. Rickard (Ed.), *Behavioral interventions in human problems* (pp. 201–22). New York: Pergamon Press.

McMurrin, S.M. (1967, January 14). What tasks for the schools? *Saturday Review,* 40–3.

Mechanical teacher aids 3-Rs. (1954, June 29). *Boston Globe.*

Metzl, J.M. (2003). *Prozac on the couch: Prescribing gender in the era of wonder drugs.* Durham and London: Duke University Press.

Meyerson, L., Kerr, N., and Michael, J. (1967). Behavior modification in rehabilitation. In S. Bijou and D. Baer (Eds.), *Child development: Readings in experimental analysis* (pp. 214–39). New York: Appleton-Century-Crofts.

Michael, J.L. (1975). Quality control in a profession. In W.S. Wood (Ed.), *Issues in evaluating behavior modification: Proceedings of the First Drake conference on professional issues in behavior analysis* (pp. 187–91). Champaign, IL: Research Press.

– (2003). Science and human behavior: A tutorial in behavior analysis. *Journal of the Experimental Analysis of Behavior, 80,* 321–8.

– (2004, June 1). Interview with the author, Boston, MA.

Milan, M.A., and McKee, J.M. (1976). The cellblock token economy: Token reinforcement procedures in a maximum security correctional institution for adult male felons. *Journal of Applied Behavior Analysis, 9,* 253–75.

Miller, G.A. (1969). Psychology as a means of promoting human welfare. *American Psychologist, 24,* 1063–75.

Miller, H.L. (1983). More than promissory? Reflections on the once and future experimental analysis of human behavior. *Psychological Record, 33,* 551–64.

Mills, J.A. (1998). *Control: A history of behavioral psychology.* New York: New York University Press.

Miracle gadget makes boys like arithmetic. (1954, June 29). *Boston Herald*, 1, 3.

Misplaced zeal. (1972, January 1). *New Republic*, 14.

Monahan, J. (1977, June). Prisons: A wary verdict on rehabilitation. *APA Monitor*, 8, 13.

Moore, J. (2008). *Conceptual foundations of radical behaviorism*. Cornwell-on-Hudson, NY: Sloan.

Moos, R., and Brownstein, R. (1977). *Environment and utopia: A synthesis*. New York: Plenum Press.

Morawski, J. (1982). Assessing psychology's moral heritage through our neglected utopias. *American Psychologist*, 37, 1082–95.

Morisse, D., Batra, L., Hess, L., Silverman, R., and Corrigan, P. (1996). A demonstration of a token economy for the real world. *Applied and Preventive Psychology*, 5, 41–6.

Morris, E.K. (1993). Behavior analysis and mechanism: One is not the other. *Behavior Analyst*, 16, 25–43.

Morris, E.K., and Smith, N.G. (2003). Bibliographic processes and products, and a bibliography of the published primary-source works of B.F. Skinner. *Behavior Analyst*, 26, 41–67.

Morris, E.K., Smith, N.G., and Altus, D.E. (2005). B.F. Skinner's contributions to applied behaviour analysis. *Behavior Analyst*, 28, 99–131.

National Commission for the Protection of Human Subjects of Biomedical and Behavioral Research. (1976). *Report and recommendations: Research involving prisoners*. DHEW Publication No. (OS) 76–131. Washington, DC: U.S. Government Printing Office.

O'Donnell, J.M. (1985). *The origins of behaviorism: American psychology, 1870–1920*. New York: New York University Press.

O'Donohue. W.J., Henderson, D.A., Hayes, S.C., Fisher, J.E., and Hayes, L.J. (Eds.) (2001). *A history of the behavioral therapies: Founders' personal histories*. Reno, NV: Context Press.

O'Leary, K.D., and Becker, W.C. (1967). Behavior modification of an adjustment class: A token reinforcement program. *Exceptional Children*, 33, 637–42.

Packer, R.E. (1963, May). Tomorrow: Automated schools. *Science Digest*, 34–8.

Palmer, D.C. (2006). On Chomsky's appraisal of Skinner's *Verbal Behavior*. A half century of misunderstanding. *Behavior Analyst*, 29, 253–67.

Paul, G.L., and Lentz, R.J. (1977). *Psychosocial treatment of chronic mental patients:Milieu versus social learning programs*. Cambridge, MA: Harvard University Press.

Pearce, D. (1972, August). God is a variable interval. *Playboy*, 81–6, 170, 172, 174, 176.

Peterson, M.E. (1978). The Midwestern Association of Behavior Analysis: Past, present, future. *Behavior Analyst*, 1, 3–15.

Phillips, E.L. (1968). Achievement Place: Token reinforcement procedures in a home-style rehabilitation setting for 'pre-delinquent' boys. *Journal of Applied Behavior Analysis, 1,* 213–23.

Pickren, W.E. (2000). A whisper of salvation: American psychologists and religion in the popular press, 1884–1908. *American Psychologist, 55,* 1022–4.

Prilleltensky, I. (1989). Psychology and the status quo. *American Psychologist, 44,* 795–802.

– (1994). On the social legacy of B.F. Skinner: Rhetoric of change, philosophy of adjustment. *Theory and Psychology, 4,* 125–37.

Professional issues in behavior analysis. (1974, July). *Division 25 Recorder, 9(2),* 10–11.

Programed learning. (1961, March 24). *Time, 36,* 38.

Pryor, K. (1999). *Don't shoot the dog: The new art of teaching and training.* New York: Bantam.

Reinhold, R. (1972, April 21). B.F. Skinner's philosophy fascist? Depends on how it's used, he says. *New York Times,* 41.

Rice, B. (1968, March 17). Skinner agrees he is the most important influence in psychology. *New York Times Magazine,* 27, 85, 87–8, 90, 95, 98, 108, 110, 112, 114.

Richards, G. (1996). *Putting psychology in its place: An introduction from a critical historical perspective.* London and New York: Routledge.

Richelle, M. (1993). *B.F. Skinner: A reappraisal.* Hillsdale, NJ: Erlbaum.

Ridgeway, J. (1966, June 4). Computer-tutor. *New Republic,* 19–22.

Risley, T. (1975). Certify procedures not people. In W.S. Wood (Ed.), *Issues in evaluating behavior modification: Proceedings of the First Drake conference on professional issues in behavior analysis* (pp. 159–81). Champaign, IL: Research Press.

– (2001). Do good, take data. In W.J. O'Donohue, D.A. Henderson, S.C. Hayes, J.E. Fisher, and L.J. Hayes (Eds.), *A history of the behavioral therapies:Founders' personal histories* (pp. 267–87). Reno, NV: Context Press.

– (2005). Montrose M. Wolf (1935–2004). Unpublished manuscript in the possession of the author.

Robinson, J. (1996). Comunidad Los Horcones: Radical behaviorism in Mexico. In B. Metcalf (Ed.), *Shared visions, shared lives: Communal living around the globe* (pp. 142–53). Findhorn, Scotland: Findhorn Press.

Robinson, P. (1983). Psychology's scrambled egos. *Washington Post Book World, 13(28),* 5–7.

Roediger, R. (2004, March). What happened to behaviorism. *APS Observer, 7(3),* 1–5.

Rose, N. (1992). Engineering the human soul: Analyzing psychological expertise. *Science in Context, 5,* 351–69.

– (1996). *Inventing our-selves: Psychology, power, and personhood.* New York and Cambridge: Cambridge University Press.

Rosen, G. (1976). The development and use of non-prescription behavior therapies. *American Psychologist, 31,* 139–41.

Rouse, J. (1987). *Knowledge and power: Toward a political philosophy of science.* Ithaca, NY: Cornell University Press.

Ruckmich, C.A. (1918). Pseudo-psychology. *Science, 48* (new series), 191–3.

Ruiz, M.R. (1995). B.F. Skinner's radical behaviourism: Historical misconstructions and grounds for feminist reconstructions. *Psychology of Women Quarterly, 19,* 161–79.

Rutherford, A. (2000). Radical behaviorism and psychology's public: B.F. Skinner in the popular press, 1934–1990. *History of Psychology, 3,* 371–95.

– (2003). B.F. Skinner's technology of behavior in American life: From consumer culture to counterculture. *Journal of the History of the Behavioral Sciences, 39,* 1–23.

– (2004). A 'visible scientist': B.F. Skinner writes for the popular press. *European Journal of Behavior Analysis, 5,* 109–20.

– (2005). B.F. Skinner. In John Shook (Ed.), *Dictionary of modern American philosophers* (pp. 2228–34). Bristol: Thoemmes Continuum.

– (2006). The social control of behavior control: Behavior modification, *Individual Rights,* and research ethics in America, 1971–1979. *Journal of the History of the Behavioral Sciences, 42,* 203–20.

Sanford, R. (1977, March 27). Utopia isn't what it used to be. *St. Louis Post Dispatch,* 21.

Sarason, S.B. (1974). *The psychological sense of community: Prospects for a community psychology.* San Francisco: Jossey-Bass.

Schaefer, H.H., and Martin, P.L. (1966). Behavioral therapy for 'apathy' of hospitalized schizophrenics. *Psychological Reports, 19,* 1147–58.

Schneider, S.M., and Morris, E.K. (1987). A history of the term *radical behaviourism* from Watson to Skinner. *Behavior Analyst, 10,* 27–39.

Schur, C. (1946, March 4). Mechanical baby-tender saves mother time. *Toronto star.*

Segal, E.F. (1987). Walden Two: The morality of anarchy. *Behavior Analyst, 10,* 147–60.

Seligman, D. (1958, October). The low productivity of the education industry. *Fortune,* 135–8, 195–6.

Sennett, R. (1971, October 24). [Review of the book *Beyond freedom and Dignity.*] *New York Times Book Review,* 1, 12, 14, 16, 18.

Shapin, S., and Schaffer, S. (1985). *Leviathan and the air pump: Hobbes, Boyle, and the experimental life.* Princeton, NJ: Princeton University Press.

Shook, G.L., and Neisworth, J.T. (2005). Ensuring appropriate qualifications for applied behavior analyst professionals: The Behavior Analyst Certification Board. *Exceptionality, 13,* 3–10.

Sidman, M. (2004). EAHB-SIG Distinguished Career Award address, Association for Behavior Analysis International 30th Annual Convention, Boston, MA.

Silberman, C.E. (1966, August). Technology is knocking at the schoolhouse door. *Fortune*, 120–5, 198, 203–5.

Skinner, B.F. (1938). *The behavior of organisms: An experimental analysis*. New York: Appleton-Century.

– (1945, October). Baby in a box – introducing the mechanical baby tender. *Ladies Home Journal*, 62, 30–1, 135–6, 138.

– (1948). *Walden two*. New York: Macmillan.

– (1950). Are theories of learning necessary? *Psychological Review*, 57, 193–216.

– (1953). *Science and human behavior*. New York: Macmillan.

– (1954). The science of learning and the art of teaching. *Harvard Educational Review*, 24, 86–97.

– (1958). Teaching machines. *Science*, 128, 969–77.

– (1960). Pigeons in a pelican. *American Psychologist*, 15, 28–37.

– (1961a). The design of cultures. *Daedulus*, 90, 534–46.

– (1961b). Teaching machines, *Scientific American*, 205, 90–102.

– (1971a). *Beyond freedom and dignity*. New York: Knopf.

– (1971b). Foreword. In H.L. Cohen and J. Filipczak, *A new learning environment* (pp. xvii-xviii). San Francisco: Jossey-Bass.

– (1971c, February 5). What I said at the Festschrift dinner (plus a few things I forgot to say and a few I wish I had). Unpublished remarks. Copy with the author.

– (1976). *Particulars of my life*. New York: Knopf.

– (1979). *The shaping of a behaviorist*. New York: Knopf.

– (1980). *Notebooks, B.F. Skinner*. Englewood Cliffs, NJ: Prentice-Hall Inc.

– (1981). Charles B. Ferster – a personal memoir. *Journal of the Experimental Analysis of Behavior*, 35, 259–61.

– (1983a). *A matter of consequences*. New York: Knopf.

– (1983b, September). Origins of a behaviorist. *Psychology Today*, 22–33.

– (2004/1968). Psychology in the year 2000. *Journal of the Experimental Analysis of Behavior*, 81, 207–13.

Skinner, B.F., Solomon, H., and Lindsley, O.R. (1954). A new method for the experimental analysis of the behavior of psychotic patients. *Journal of Nervous and Mental Disease*, 120, 403–6.

Skinner, B.F., and Vaughan, M.E. (1983). *Enjoy old age*. New York: Norton.

Slater, L. (2004). *Opening Skinner's box: Great psychological experiments of the twentieth century*. New York: Norton.

Smith, L.D. (1992). On prediction and control: B.F. Skinner and the technological ideal of science. *American Psychologist*, 47, 216–23.

– (1996a). Knowledge as power: The Baconian roots of Skinner's social melior-ism. In L.D. Smith and W.R. Woodward (Eds.), *B.F. Skinner and behaviorism in American culture* (pp. 56–82). Bethlehem, PA: Lehigh University Press.

– (1996b). Situating B.F. Skinner and behaviorism in American culture. In L.D. Smith and W.R. Woodward (Eds.), *B.F. Skinner and behaviorism in American culture* (pp. 294–315). Bethlehem, PA: Lehigh University Press.

Smith, R. (1997). *The Norton history of the human sciences.* New York: Norton.

Sokolov, R. (1978, December). Thinner with Skinner. *Cosmopolitan,* 128, 130, 192.

Spigel, L. (1992). *Make room for TV: Television and the family ideal in postwar Amer-ica.* Chicago: University of Chicago Press.

Staats, A.W., Staats, C.K., Schultz, R.E., and Wolf, M.M. (1962). The condition-ing of textual responses using 'extrinsic' reinforcers. *Journal of the Experimental Analysis of Behavior,* 5, 33–40.

Stenger, C.A., and Peck, C.P. (1970). Token-economy programs in the Veterans Administration. *Hospital and Community Psychiatry,* 21, 39–43.

Stevens, W.K. (1971, September 3). In behaviorist's ideal state, control replaces liberty. *New York Times,* 29.

Stockdill, J.W. (2005). National mental health policy and the community mental health centers, 1963–1981. In W.E. Pickren and S.F. Schneider (Eds.), *Psychology and the national institute of mental health: A historical analysis of science, practice, and policy* (pp. 261–93). Washington, DC: American Psychological Association.

Stolz, S.B., and Associates. (1978). *Ethical issues in behavior modification: Report of the American Psychological Association Commission.* San Francisco: Jossey-Bass.

Stolz, S.B., Wienckowski, L.A., and Brown, B.S. (1975). Behavior modification: A perspective on critical issues. *American Psychologist,* 30, 1027–48.

Stuart, R.B. (1967). Behavioral control of overeating. *Behaviour Research and Therapy,* 5, 357–65.

Stuart, R.B., and Davis, B. (1972). *Slim chance in a fat world: Behavioral control of obesity.* Champaign, IL: Research Press.

Sulzer-Azaroff, B., Thaw, J., and Thomas, C. (1975). Behavioral competencies for the evaluation of behavior modifiers. In W.S. Wood (Ed.), *Issues in evaluat-ing behavior modification: Proceedings of the First Drake conference on professional issues in behavior analysis* (pp. 47–98). Champaign, IL: Research Press.

Suppes, P. (1967, January 14). The computer and excellence. *Saturday Review,* 46, 48, 50.

Sutherland, A. (2008). *What Shamu taught me about life, love, and marriage: Lessons for people from animals and their trainers.* New York: Random House.

Teaching by machine. (1954, July 17). *Science News Letter,* 38.

Thoresen, C.E., and Mahoney, M.J. (1974). *Behavioral self-control.* New York: Holt, Rinehart, and Winston.

Todd. J.T. (1996). A history of Division 25 (Experimental analysis of behavior). In D.A. Dewsbury (Ed.), *Unification through division: Histories of the divisions of the APA, Vol. 1* (pp. 157–93). Washington, DC: APA.

Todd, J.T., and Morris, E.K. (1983). Misconception and miseducation: Presentations of radical behaviorism in psychology textbooks. *Behavior Analyst, 6,* 153–60.

Trotter, S. (1974, August). ACLU scores token economy. *APA Monitor, 5,* 5.

Trotter, S., and Warren, J. (1974, April). Behavior modification under fire. *APA Monitor, 5,* 1 1.

Twyman, J.S. (2007). A new era of science and practice in behavior analysis. *Association for Behavior Analysis International Newsletter, 30(3),* 1–4.

Ubell, E. (1954, June 29). Machine teaches kids arithmetic painlessly. *New York Herald Tribune.*

Ulmer, R.A. (1976). *On the development of a token economy mental hospital treatment program.* New York: Wiley.

Ulrich, R. (1967). Behavior control and public concern. *Psychological Record, 17,* 229–34.

Updates from ABA's affiliated chapters (2007). *Association for Behavior Analysis International Newsletter, 30(2),* 19–39.

Utopia or disaster. (1983, January). *Science Digest,* 14, 15, 104, 106.

van Sommers, P. (1962). Oxygen-motivated behavior in the goldfish, Carassius auratus. *Science, 137,* 678–9.

Vargas, E.A., and Vargas, J.S. (1996). B.F. Skinner and the origins of programmed instruction. In L.D. Smith and W.R. Woodward (Eds.), *B.F. Skinner and behaviorism in American culture* (pp. 237–53). Bethlehem, PA: Lehigh University Press.

Vargas, J.S. (2000, March 3). Interview with author, Morgantown, WV.

Virués-Ortega, J. (2006). The case against B.F. Skinner 45 years later: An encounter with Noam Chomsky. *Behavior Analyst, 29,* 243–52.

Wald, S. (2005, June). Making room for mentalism: Limits of the neo-behaviorist regime in American experimental psychology, 1938–1955. Paper presented at the 37th Annual Meeting of Cheiron, The International Society for the History of the Social and Behavioral Sciences, Berkeley, CA.

Walker, J. (1993). *Couching resistance: Women, film, and psychoanalytic psychiatry.* Minneapolis: University of Minnesota Press.

Ward, S.C. (2002). *Modernizing the mind: Psychological knowledge and the remaking of society.* Westport, CT: Praeger.

Warren, J. (1974, April). Pot-pourri. *APA Monitor, 5,* 3.

Watson, D.L., and Tharp, R.G. (1972). *Self-directed behaviour: Self-modification for personal adjustment.* Monterey, CA: Brooks/Cole Publishing Company.

Watson, J.B. (1928). *Psychological care of infant and child.* New York: Norton.

Weiner, H. (1962). Some effects of response cost upon human operant behavior. *Journal of the Experimental Analysis of Behavior, 5,* 201–8.

– (1963). Response cost and the aversive control of human operant behavior. *Journal of the Experimental Analysis of Behavior, 6,* 415–21.

Weizmann, F. (2005). [Review of Slater's *Opening Skinner's box: Great psychological experiments of the twentieth century.*] *Journal of the History of the Behavioral Sciences, 41,* 402–4.

Wesolowski, M.D. (2002). Pioneer profiles: A few minutes with Sid Bijou. *Behavior Analyst, 25,* 15–27.

What makes a researcher 'good copy.' (1975, August). *APA Monitor, 6,* 1, 8.

What's happening in education? (1967, September). *Today's Health,* 47–55.

Whitley, R. (1985). Knowledge producers and knowledge acquirers: Popularization as a relation between scientific fields and their publics. In T. Shinn and R. Whitley (Eds.), *Expository science: Forms and functions of popularization* (pp. 3–30). Dordrecht: D. Reidel Publishing Company.

Wiener, D.N. (1996). *B.F. Skinner: Benign anarchist.* Boston: Allyn and Bacon.

Winett, R.A., and Winkler, R.C. (1972). Current behavior modification in the classroom: Be still, be quiet, be docile. *Journal of Applied Behavior Analysis, 5,* 499–504.

Winkler, R.C. (1970). Management of chronic psychiatric patients by a token reinforcement system. *Journal of Applied Behavior Analysis, 3,* 47–55.

Wolf, M.M. (1993). Remembrances of issues past: Celebrating *JABA*'s 25th anniversary. *Journal of Applied Behavior Analysis, 26,* 543–4.

– (2001). Application of operant conditioning procedures to the behavior problems of an autistic child: A 25-year follow-up and the development of the teaching family model. In W.J. O'Donohue, D.A. Henderson, S.C. Hayes, J.E. Fisher, and L.J. Hayes (Eds.), *A history of the behavioral therapies: Founders' personal histories* (pp. 289–94). Reno, NV: Context Press.

Wolf, M.M., Risley, T.R., Johnston, M.K., Harris, F.R., and Allen, K.E. (1967). Application of operant conditioning procedures to the behavior problems of an autistic child: A follow-up and extension. *Behavior Research and Therapy, 5,* 103–11.

Wolf, M.M., Risley, T.R., and Mees, H. (1964). Application of operant conditioning procedures to the behavior problems of the autistic child. *Behavior Research and Therapy, 1,* 305–12.

Wood, W.S. (Ed.). (1975a). *Issues in evaluating behavior modification: Proceedings of the First Drake conference on professional issues in behavior analysis.* Champaign, IL: Research Press.

– (1975b). What is 'applied' in the applied analysis of behavior? In W.S. Wood (Ed.), *Issues in evaluating behavior modification: Proceedings of the First Drake conference on professional issues in behavior analysis* (pp. 23–38). Champaign, IL: Research Press.

Woodward, W.R. (1996). Skinner and behaviorism as cultural icons: From local knowledge to reader reception. In L.D. Smith and W.R. Woodward (Eds.), *B.F. Skinner and behaviorism in American culture* (pp. 7–29). Bethlehem, PA: Lehigh University Press.

Wyatt, W.J. (1993, Summer). Myths and misperceptions about Skinner studied. *Behavior Analysis Digest, 5(2)*, 1.

Yafa, S. (1973, March). Zap, you're normal. *Playboy*, 87, 90, 184–8.

Zuriff, G.E. (1979). The demise of behaviourism – exaggerated rumor? [Review of Mackenzie's *Behaviorism and the limits of scientific method.*] *Journal of the Experimental Analysis of Behavior, 32*, 129–36.

– (1980). Radical behaviourist epistemology. *Psychological Bulletin, 87*, 337–50.

– (1985). *Behaviorism: A conceptual reconstruction.* New York: Columbia University Press.

Index